THE AUTHOR

Rosemary Conley lives in Leicestershire with her husband, Mike Rimmington, with whom she runs Rosemary Conley Enterprises and Rosemary Conley Diet and Fitness Clubs Ltd.

A qualified exercise teacher, Rosemary has worked in the field of slimming and exercise for twenty years, but it was in 1986 that she discovered by accident that low-fat eating led to a leaner body. Forced on to a very low-fat diet as a result of a gallstone problem, not only did Rosemary avoid major surgery but her previously disproportionately large hips and thighs reduced dramatically in size. After extensive research and trials her *Hip and Thigh Diet* was published in 1988 by Arrow Books. This book and its sequel, *Rosemary Conley's Complete Hip and Thigh Diet*, have dominated the bestseller lists for five years and have sold in excess of two million copies. Rosemary Conley's *Hip and Thigh Diet* has been translated into five languages, including Hebrew and Greek. Subsequent titles, *Hip and Thigh Diet Cookbook, 1 & 2* (written with chef and cookery writer Patricia Bourne), *Inch Loss Plan*, *Metabolism Booster Diet* and *Whole Body Programme*, have all been instant number 1 bestsellers.

Rosemary has travelled the world promoting her books and has made numerous appearances on national and international television and radio. Since 1990 she has presented her own diet and fitness series on network television. Rosemary's *Whole Body Programme* video was published in January 1991 and this topped the general video bestseller chart for several months. Still the biggest-selling fitness video in the UK, Rosemary received a double platinum disc to commemorate sales exceeding 300,000. Further videos have included *Whole Body Programme 2, 7-Day Workout* and her *Top to Toe Collection*. Her latest video, *Whole Body Programme 3 – Aerobics and Beyond*, was released in January 1993.

SHAPE UP
FOR SUMMER

The 14-Day Whole Body Action Plan

Rosemary Conley

ARROW

First published in Arrow 1993

7 9 10 8 6

© Rosemary Conley Enterprises 1993

The right of Rosemary Conley to be identified as the author
of this work has been asserted by her in accordance
with the Copyright, Designs and Patents Act, 1988

Arrow Books Limited
Random House UK Ltd, 20 Vauxhall Bridge Road, London SW1V 2SA

Random House Australia (Pty) Limited
20 Alfred Street, Milsons Point, Sydney,
New South Wales 2061, Australia

Random House New Zealand Limited
18 Poland Road, Glenfield
Auckland 10, New Zealand

Random House South Africa (Pty) Limited
PO Box 337, Bergvlei, South Africa

Random House UK Limited Reg. No. 954009

A CIP catalogue record for this book
is available from the British Library

Papers used by Random House UK Limited
are natural, recyclable products made from wood grown in
sustainable forests. The manufacturing processes conform to
the environmental regulations of the country of origin.

ISBN 0 09 923101 8

Printed and bound in Great Britain by
Cox & Wyman Ltd, Reading, Berkshire

WARNING

If you have a medical condition, or are pregnant, the diet and
exercises described in this book should not be followed without first consulting your doctor. All guidelines and warnings
should be read carefully, and the author and publisher cannot accept responsibility for injuries or damage arising out of
a failure to comply with the same.

Contents

PART III
Summer At Home

Introduction

With the arrival of a gloriously warm and sunny day many of us experience a real panic as we slip into last year's sleeveless dress, or, even worse, the dreaded shorts. Not only do the clothes appear to have shrunk during winter storage, but the body appears to have gone completely to seed. The arms are pale and saggy and, horror of horrors, the legs look like whitewashed trees trunks!

We hurriedly remove the summer gear and slip back into a lightweight winter number and decide to sweat it out for the rest of the day under camouflage of sleeves, slacks and anti-perspirant. But how long can this go on for?

In this book, I have created a special 14-day Shape-Up for Summer diet and exercise programme and have included a number of tips and ideas for making the most of ourselves on the beach and for keeping any damage to the diet to a minimum while on holiday. There's advice on coping with travel stress, bed-and-breakfast, self-catering and hotel holidays, as well as a three-day post-holiday corrector diet to repair any damage that's been done. In addition, I have given a whole range of suggestions for healthy-eating at home during the summer – from picnics to barbecues.

If you have a lot of weight to shed, don't leave it until two weeks before you go away to start dieting. Begin at least a month beforehand so that the weight you lose is real fat that burns away and not just a temporary fluid reduction which makes you weigh less.

However, whether you have a lot or a little weight to lose, or perhaps want to stay as you are but be healthy, what you eat is crucial. 'We are what we eat' is absolutely right and if we want a beautiful healthy body that will serve us for a long and happy life, we need to eat good, healthy food and take regular exercise.

Human beings are a strange race. When we drive a car we make certain that it has enough oil in the engine, that the battery is topped up with distilled water, that the various parts are sufficiently greased and that we put good quality petrol in the tank. We also keep an eye on the tyres to make sure they don't go flat and wear out prematurely and we keep the bodywork clean so that it won't deteriorate or look old before its time. We also spend significant sums of money putting our car in for a regular service to make sure that it is kept in good order and will be reliable. We spend all this time, energy and money because if the car broke down it would be extremely inconvenient. But do we spend as much time and trouble caring about our own body? Do we go to the doctor every six months for a blood pressure check, do we ever stop to think whether the food we eat and drink is actually good for us? Do we seriously consider how incredibly inconvenient it would be for us, and our family, if we were ill? I am sure we all know the answer to these questions, but isn't it ironic that we put our own health and fitness so low on the list of priorities of life? We are usually more careful about feeding our *pets* correctly and giving *them* regular exercise than we are about caring for ourselves!

From now on I would like you to treat your body with the same loving care and attention that you would give to a brand-new car, the car of your dreams, your pride and joy. Would you like to feel that at the end of a few weeks your *own body* will be your pride and joy? Together we *can* transform you, from being tired and listless, flabby, overweight and lacking in self-confidence, into a *happy new you*! After the two-week diet and exercise programme, any-one who still has excess weight and inches (cm) to lose should just stick with it and continue the diet by selecting any of the menus and keeping up the daily exercises. Body reshaping has never been simpler.

This book is designed for the whole family to enjoy healthy, tasty and satisfying meals, with the option for those not trying to lose any weight to eat all they need in order to maintain their energy requirements during the summer months.

Let this summer be a summer to remember as the time you 'rediscovered' your body and found new youth and energy.

PART I

14-Day Shape-Up For Summer Diet and Whole Body Action Plan

1

14-Day Diet and Fat-Burner Fitness Programme

On the following pages you will find a 14-day diet and fat-burner exercise plan comprising a daily menu and a daily aerobic workout. The menus and workouts have both been designed to effect the maximum weight loss in the minimum time in preparation for your holiday.

Within each day of this programme I have included some encouraging words to help you stick to the diet and persevere with the exercises. If you follow the diet and exercise plans as directed, you will be amazed how much weight you can lose and how many inches (cm) will disappear in this short 14-day period.

Before you begin the 14-day diet I want you to be quite certain that you are going to be committed for the duration. If you are half-hearted about it, you will almost certainly fail. If you are totally determined, you will almost certainly succeed. During these 14 days I am asking you not to eat anything between meals, not to cheat at all, to refrain from eating anything that is listed on the **Forbidden List** (see page 20), and to make a space in each day to do your aerobic exercises.

The daily menus have been designed to incorporate all the necessary nutrients as well as a sufficient volume of food to satisfy you. If the menus that I have suggested are inconvenient, inappropriate or simply not to your liking, then turn to the 14-Day Free Choice diet which is detailed in Chapter 2. From this you can select any breakfast, lunch, dinner and dessert option. These can be used in place of any of the dishes suggested within the day-by-day Shape-Up for Summer diet. For a diet to be successful it has to work for you. I hope you will be able to work out *your* diet to your absolute liking – so that you won't actually feel that you are dieting, but more that you are eating for health and that the loss of weight and inches (cm) is a tremendous bonus.

Just prior to going on holiday we often feel that we are at the end of our tether. I can remember saying on more than one occasion, 'It's a good job we're going on holiday next week – I feel I just couldn't cope any longer!' I'm quite sure that such feelings are totally psychological but, nevertheless, the prospect of glorious sunshine, a beautiful suntan and a break from our normal world does seem incredibly inviting. If we feel good about our body prior to going away, there is no doubt that we will cope much better with the run-up to the holiday because we will be happier in ourselves and looking forward to getting on to the beach – or wherever – rather than dreading it!

So, here is your opportunity to lose several pounds (kg) and inches (cm) and get your body into a healthy, tip-top condition ready for sun, sea and relaxation.

All the meals are calorie-counted and contain the minimum of fat, but they incorporate sufficient essential fatty acids and lots of fibre in order to promote optimum nutrition. The high-fibre content will encourage elimination of waste products, thus leaving our body healthier.

The daily exercise programme includes a 'fat-burner workout' which is exactly what it says. Aerobic exercise helps us to burn away fat and these carefully designed sequences incorporate the many elements to ensure an effective and safe aerobic workout. Our body burns fat when we work out aerobically at a level that makes us puff significantly, but not *so* hard that we are unable to speak. In order to achieve the level of activity at which our body actually does burn real fat from around our body, we need to ensure that the oxygen is flowing efficiently through our muscles.

It is therefore essential to make the necessary preparations included in the 'warm-up' sections to enable the oxygen to be utilized to maximum effect. In aerobic exercises oxygen gives us the energy we need to continue, but it isn't like switching on an electric light bulb. You can't just make it happen instantly. The body needs time to convert the oxygen into energy and this is done over a period of several minutes. Failure to prepare the body results in harm to the muscles and ineffective fat-burning during the workout, because that energy system has not been established. I cannot emphasize too strongly the importance of following the instructions in this exercise programme to the letter. More detailed explanations about how the workout should be followed are included on page 21. Always remember to fluctuate between 'high-' and 'low-' impact aerobics (explained later) according to your fitness level and capability.

Weigh and measure yourself before you start the diet, using a pair of scales placed on a firm board rather than carpet. Carefully note the details on the **Measurement Record Chart** on page 16. Then weigh and measure yourself again after 6 and 14 days. *Do not* weigh yourself in between.

Where appropriate, take the time and trouble to weigh items of food, as incorrect guessing can lead to diet failure. Eat sufficient at meal times to satisfy your hunger, but do not eat more than you need. It is *essential* that you eat three meals a day and if you find any of the suggested menus too filling, replace it with another that offers less bulk. All the breakfasts, lunches, dinners and desserts may be exchanged as desired. Also, if you prefer to have your main meal at lunch time and a lighter lunch menu in the evening, this is perfectly acceptable.

It is important to realize when you start this diet that you are going to have to be exceedingly strong-willed for the next 14 days. With the wonderful goal of your holiday at the end of it, you should be able to find sufficient willpower to be saintly. I do hope so. Best of luck!

Measurement Record Chart

DATE	WEIGHT	BUST	WAIST	HIPS	WIDE PART
29/6/98	11st11lb	42in	35in	41in	
6/7/98	11st 7lb	42in	34in	40in	
14/7/98	11st 6lb	41in	33	40 in	
21/7/98	11st 5lb				
28/7/98	11st 7lb	41 ½in	32	42in	
4/8/98					
29/6/98	9st 5lb	35in	30in	35½	
7/7/98	9st 3lb	34	28in	33	
14/7/98	9st 3lb	35in	28in	35½	
21/7/98	9st 2lb	34	27	35	
28/7/98	9st 6lb	34	27½	37	
4/8/98	9st 7lb	35	28	37	
11/8/98	9st 6lb	35	28	36	

TOP OF THIGHS		ABOVE KNEES		UPPER ARMS		COMMENTS
L	R	L	R	L	R	
22	22	17	6½	13	13	Mum
22	22	6½	6½	13	13	
21½	21½	16½	16½	13	13	
22	22	16	16	13	13	
21	21	15½	15½	12	11½	Fiona
21	21	15½	15½	12	11¾	
22	22	16	16	12	11½	
21½	21	15½	16	12	12	
22	22	16	16	12	12	
22	22	15½	16			
22	22	15½	15½			

DIET NOTES

Daily Allowance:

5 fl oz (125 ml) unsweetened fruit juice
10 fl oz (250 ml) skimmed or semi-skimmed milk
1 alcoholic drink per day for women
2 alcoholic drinks per day for men

Select each day:

1 Breakfast menu
1 Lunch menu
1 Dinner menu
1 Dessert menu

Weights and measures
The following conversion rates have been used throughout this book:

1 oz = 25 g; 1 fl oz = 25 ml; 1/2 pint = 250 ml.

Fruit
One piece of fresh fruit means one apple or one banana or 4 oz (100 g) any fruit such as grapes, strawberries, pineapple.

Yogurt
All yogurts should be low-fat, low-calorie varieties. Check the nutrition details on the side of the carton to make certain you choose the right one.

Sweeteners
Low-calorie artificial sweeteners may be used in place of sugar. Keep the consumption of sugar to an absolute minimum.

Bread
Bread should always be wholemeal.

Milk
Milk should be skimmed or semi-skimmed – 'silver-top' milk is acceptable providing the cream is removed.

Vegetables
'Unlimited vegetables' includes potatoes, except where they are stated separately. All vegetables must be cooked and served without fat of any kind.

Pasta
Pasta should be the egg-free variety.

Rice
Always use brown rice when possible. It is significantly more nutritious than white rice and much higher in fibre content.

Salad dressings, sauces, etc.
Recipes for Garlic Dressing, Oil-Free Vinaigrette, Marie-Rose, and Reduced-Oil Salad Dressing can be found in Chapter 13. These may be eaten freely. Branded reduced-oil salad dressings e.g. Waistline, Weight Watchers, etc., should be eaten only if included in the menus or individual recipes. However, sauces such as tomato ketchup, soy, Tabasco, Worcestershire, brown, HP, vinegar, etc. can all be eaten freely. Marmite and Bovril are also permitted. If in doubt, check the label for details of fat and calorie content.

Drinks
You should drink at least eight cups or glasses of liquid each day: water; low-calorie or diet drinks; tea and coffee (milk from daily allowance); fruit juice from daily allowance.

Tea and coffee may be drunk freely if taken black, or may be taken white provided the skimmed-milk allowance is not exceeded. Use artificial sweetener in place of sugar whenever possible.

Men may drink two alcoholic drinks per day and women one drink per day. 'One drink' means a single measure of spirits, a glass of wine, a small glass of sherry or 10 fl oz (250 ml) of beer or lager. Slimline mixers should always be used. These and diet drinks may be drunk freely.

You may drink as much water as you like. Unsweetened fruit juices, which are taken in addition to the 5 fl oz (125 ml) included in the daily allowance, should be consumed only in place of an alcoholic drink.

THE FORBIDDEN LIST

These foods are strictly forbidden (except where included in one of the recipes) whilst following the diet.

Butter, margarine, Flora, Flora Light, Gold, Gold Lowest, Outline, Delight or any similar products.
Cream, soured cream, whole milk, 'gold top' , etc.
Lard, oil (all kinds), dripping, suet, etc.
Milk puddings of any kind.
Fried foods of any kind (except dry-fried).
Fat or skin from all meats, poultry, etc.
All cheese except low-fat cottage cheese, unless otherwise stated in the diet menus.
Egg yolk (the whites may be eaten freely).
All nuts except chestnuts.
Sunflower seeds.
Goose.
All fatty meats.
Meat products, e.g. Scotch eggs, pork pie, faggots, black pudding, haggis, liver sausage, pâté.
All types of sausages and salami.

All sauces containing cream or whole milk or eggs, e.g. salad dressing, mayonnaise, French dressing, parsley sauce, cheese sauce, hollandaise sauce. (Waistline or similar dressings may only be used as stated in the diet menus.)

Cakes, sweet biscuits, pastries, sponge puddings, etc., including savoury pastries.

Chocolate, toffee, fudge, caramel, butterscotch.

Savoury biscuits and crispbreads (except Ryvita).

Lemon curd.

Marzipan.

Cocoa and cocoa products (except very low-fat brands), Horlicks.

Crisps, including low-fat crisps.

Cream soups.

Avocado pears.

Yorkshire pudding.

Egg products, e.g. quiches, egg custard, pancakes, etc.

EXPLANATORY NOTES ON THE 14-DAY FAT-BURNER WORKOUT

What do we mean by 'low-' and 'high-' impact aerobics?

The term 'low-impact' is used to describe exercises where one foot always remains on the floor (e.g. walking jog, knee raises or marching), thus reducing the impact of the raised foot as it touches the ground.

'High-impact', on the other hand, describes an exercise where both feet leave the ground at regular intervals as in jogging, jumping, skipping and so on. The impact on the feet as we land during a high-impact aerobic exercise is quite dramatic – in fact up to 10 times our body weight. Lifting our body weight off the floor at very regular intervals requires a great deal of energy. This energy is generated by the oxygen being transported by the blood to the muscles. To provide sufficient oxygen, the heart and lungs have to work much harder, thus significantly raising our heart rate and causing us to breathe faster and more deeply. It is at this level of activity that the fat-burning process is at its peak.

It is important to combine high- and low-impact aerobic exercise, allowing our body to dictate the balance between the two. Obviously, those who are considerably overweight will find high-impact exercise very taxing, not only on the heart and lungs but also on the joints. It is essential, therefore, that common sense always prevails so that over-use of muscles and excess stress on joints are prevented.

How can we make an exercise more energetic while still keeping the sequence at low-impact level?

We can make our body work harder by increasing the intensity of the movements that we are making. This can be achieved by exercising the arms at a level higher than the heart itself. Raising the arms to shoulder level and swinging them in and out, or bending and straightening them at or above shoulder level, and taking larger steps including knee lifts and so on, are all ways of increasing the intensity of an exercise. In the exercises that follow the intensity is varied by using the arms both at high and low levels. This increased intensity causes the heart to work harder as it pumps the blood around our arms against the force of gravity and therefore uses more energy. In addition, the muscles of the legs require more oxygen.

We expend the greatest amount of energy when we combine high-impact aerobic exercise with high-intensity movements. We expend significantly less energy during a workout when we are exercising at low-impact level with low-intensity movements.

Play some of your favourite lively music throughout your Fat-burner Fitness Programme. Wear suitable clothing and cushioned exercise shoes.

Do not exercise until at least 90 minutes after eating a meal.

The Mobilizing Warm-up

Important: always complete the warm-up section, including the preparatory stretches, prior to commencing the Fat-burner Workout.

The Fat-Burner Workout

Always start your Fat-burner Workout by following these exercises at low-impact level in order to thoroughly warm up your muscles and increase the flow of oxygen to them. Then repeat the Fat-burner exercises and increase the momentum and intensity of the exercises by including a jump or skip as you perform the movements, thus making them high-impact.

Alternate between high- and low-impact exercises. Your own body will tell you how energetic you should be, as this will be determined by your present fitness level.

Cooling Down

Repeat the Fat-burner exercises at low-impact level to allow your pulse rate to return to normal. Finish by repeating the stretches from the warm-up section to help bring your muscles back to normal and prevent unnecessary discomfort.

You have just 14 days in which to improve dramatically your shape and size in preparation for your well-earned summer holiday. Try to adopt a very positive attitude to your 14-day campaign and decide here and now that you are going to stick with this programme for the duration. No hesitation or wavering is allowed once you have started! Tell yourself that this time you are really going to succeed on the diet and that you are going to make time to do the exercises. If you do so, you will be thrilled with the results in just 14 days' time.

Before you even have your breakfast today, I would like you to do the following four tasks:

1 Weigh yourself on a pair of scales, wearing as little clothing as possible.
2 Measure around your bust, waist, hips, widest part, the widest part at the top of each thigh, the narrowest part above each knee, and the widest part around your upper arm. Record these measurements on the chart on page 16.
3 Try on a swimsuit or bikini that you plan to take away with you and stand in front of a full-length mirror. Take time to acknowledge how you look in the mirror today. Look at the front, side and back view if possible. Don't be put off by what you see. In just two weeks there will be a significant improvement.
4 If possible, find a skirt or pair of trousers that you will not be wearing for the next two weeks. (Something from your winter wardrobe would be ideal for this purpose.) The skirt or trousers should fit tightly on you today. Keep the garment in your summer wardrobe so that you can try it on every two or three days to measure your progress in real terms. Sometimes scales can be deceptive.

Start your day with a small glass of orange juice and enjoy your breakfast of muesli with natural yogurt. If you prefer, you could have one teaspoonful of honey instead of the sugar. Alternatively, select one of the other breakfast menus suggested in this 14-day programme or pick one from the **Free Choice Diet** in Chapter 2. Remember to stick strictly to the quantities noted.

Once you have eaten your breakfast allow your brain to register that you are to eat nothing between now and lunchtime. If at any point it says you feel hungry, dismiss such thoughts and busy yourself with a job or pastime that you enjoy. Decide at what time you are going to exercise each day and ideally stick to this same time so that you will always be able to find those essential few minutes which will make such a dramatic difference to the way you feel and look in 14 days' time. Carefully read the daily instructions for the exercise. This is very important.

If you have time, prepare the Fish Curry (*see recipe*) for this evening's meal well in advance and leave it to stand for a few hours. The spices will then have a chance to penetrate deeply into the fish and make an even tastier meal.

All recipes are included in Chapter 13 and can be easily located by referring to the index of recipes at the back of this book.

Have a great day and look forward to a disciplined but highly rewarding 14 days and a very happy new you at the end of it.

DAY 1 FAT-BURNER FITNESS PROGRAMME

Mobilizing Warm-up

1. Shoulder rotations
Rotate alternate shoulders
backwards 8 times and forwards
8 times (4 each shoulder). Then
repeat, rotating both shoulders
together.

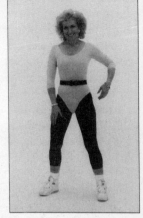

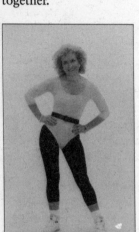

2. Alternate hip rotations
Rotate hips first in a clockwise
direction, then in an anti-
clockwise direction. Repeat
alternate hip rotations 8 times (4
each direction).

3. Alternate heel digs, arm flexes
Do 24 heel digs (12 each heel),
alternating heels and at the same
time flexing and straightening
the arm

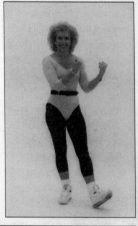

4. *Sideways curve*
Do 16 sideways curves to alternate sides (8 each side).

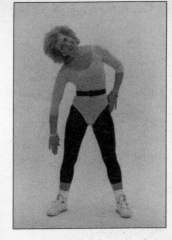

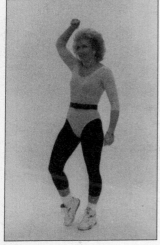

5. *Walking jog, arm circles*
Do a walking jog on the spot, circling alternate arms backwards as you step. Do 16 circles (8 each arm).

6. *Waist twist*
With knees slightly bent and elbows bent outwards at shoulder level, twist upper body to alternate sides. Do 16 (8 each side).

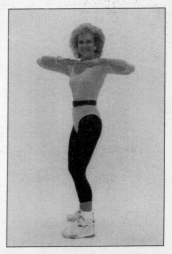

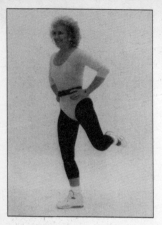

7. *Kick back*
Kick back with alternate feet, bending the knee as you kick. Do 16 (8 each foot).

Stretches

8. *Front thigh stretch*
Stand with feet together. Bend left leg and take hold of its foot with left hand as shown. Ease foot as close to seat as you can and hold for 8 counts. Slowly release and repeat with other leg.

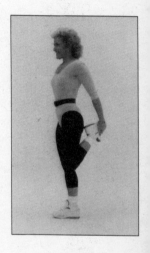

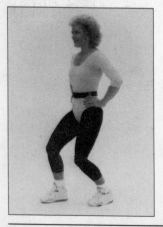

9. *Calf stretch*
Stand as shown with feet parallel, one foot in front of the other. Keeping both heels on the floor, bend both knees and hold for 8 counts. Slowly release, and repeat with other leg in front.

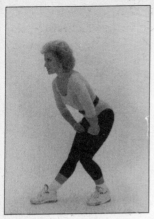

10. *Hamstring stretch*
Stand with feet parallel and hip-width apart, one foot in front of the other. Keep front leg straight and bend the knee of the other leg as shown, ensuring that both heels remain on the floor. Hold for 8 counts. Slowly release, and repeat with the other leg in front.

11. *Inner thigh stretch*
Stand with feet wide apart with one foot turned out to the side slightly and the knee bent directly over that foot. Keep the other leg straight and foot parallel. Hold for 8 counts. Slowly release, change legs and repeat.

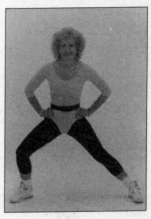

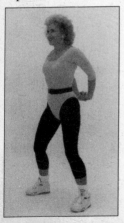

12. *Chest stretch*
Stand with feet a comfortable distance apart and knees slightly bent. Extend arms behind you and, clasping the hands, raise arms as high as possible. Hold for 8 counts.

13. *Waist stretch*
Stand with feet a comfortable distance apart, one hand on hip. Reach other arm over to side with palm of hand facing ceiling. Hold for 8 counts. Slowly release, and repeat to the other side.

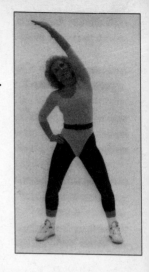

Pulse-Raiser Warm-up

Follow exercises 14–20 at low-impact level.

14. *Marching*
March on the spot. Do 32 steps.

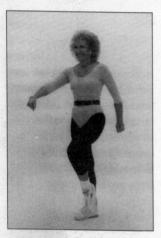

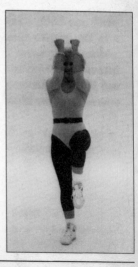

15. *Knee raises, arms out and in*
Raise alternate knees, bringing bent arms out and in at shoulder level. Do 16 knee raises (8 each knee).

16. *Step and kick*
Step with one foot and kick across with the other foot, swinging arms to opposite side. Do 16 to alternate sides (8 each side).

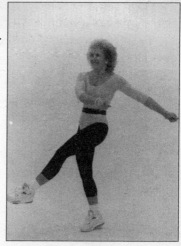

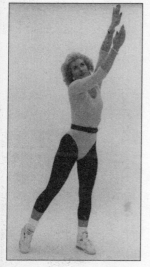

17. *Arm swinging*
Swing arms from side to side, bending the knees and transferring weight from one foot to the other as you go. Do 16 (8 each side).

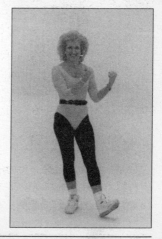

18. *Alternate heel digs, arm flexes*
Do 16 heel digs (8 each heel), alternating heels and flexing and straightening the arms.

19. Kick back

Kick back with alternate feet, bending the knee as you kick and, at the same time, swinging arms out to sides and then crossing them in front. Do 16 (8 each foot).

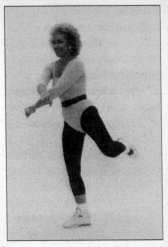

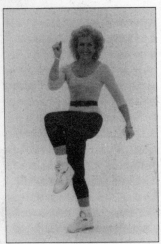

20. Knee raises to opposite elbow

Raise alternate knees towards opposite elbow. Do 16 (8 each knee).

Fat-Burner Workout

Repeat exercises 15–20 at high-impact level (or low-impact as necessary), then proceed to exercise 21 performing it at high-impact level.

21. Sideways jogging

Jog from side to side. Do 16 (8 each side).

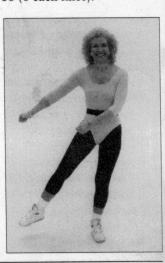

22. *Step and point*

Extend one leg out to the side, pointing the foot, and at the same time swing arms out to the sides. Bring leg and arms in again, and repeat to the other side. Do 16 (8 each side).

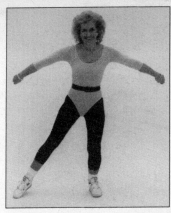

Cool Down

Repeat exercises 14–20 and 22 at low-impact level.

Repeat stretches 8–13.

DAY 1 DIET

Breakfast
1 oz (25 g) muesli mixed with 5 oz (125 g) natural yogurt, plus 1 teaspoon sugar.

Lunch
2 slices (2 oz/50 g) bread spread with Reduced-Oil Salad Dressing (*see recipe*), filled with salad and 3 oz (75 g) tuna (in brine) mixed with 2 teaspoons Reduced-Oil Salad Dressing (*see recipe*).

Dinner
Fish Curry (*see recipe*) with 6 oz (150 g) boiled brown rice (cooked weight), plus Minty Melon and Yogurt Salad (*see recipe*). Select any dessert from page 175.

I hope you enjoyed yesterday's menus and that you are feeling confident and positive about your ability to stick with this programme for another 13 days.

I also hope you found the exercises enjoyable and managed to follow the instructions so that you were able to work out with optimum benefit to your body. As the days progress, I am sure you will find the exercises easier and you will be surprised at how much energy you find developing. Don't be tempted to do too much too soon at high-impact level, but as the days go past feel free to increase the amount of energy you put into your workout.

In preparation for your holiday and the suntan that you are no doubt hoping to acquire, start to put oil in your daily bath and apply body lotion all over your body after every bath or shower. Do these every day until you go away and continue during and after your holiday. Keeping the skin moisturized encourages an even tan and helps to keep the skin supple, preventing burning. Continuing to apply body lotion after the holiday will also help to prevent peeling if you do happen to get burnt in any area. (See **Body Care** chapter for further details and advice.)

Now is the time to begin preparing the clothes that you intend to pack for your holiday. Start selecting your outfits and co-ordinate them to achieve maximum versatility. Don't buy any new clothes until you have decided exactly which colour you wish to match with whatever is already in your existing summer wardrobe. If you need sun protection creams, now is the time to purchase them so that you can try them out to ensure you do not experience an allergic reaction. If you do, there is time to recover before you go away. Remember an allergic reaction can be greatly minimized by taking an anti-histamine tablet which is available over the counter at your chemist. Keep some of these to take on holiday too. They can dramatically reduce the effect of an insect bite and should always be carried with you if you are going to a hot or tropical climate.

Tonight's dinner menu offers Chicken with Orange and Apricots (*see recipe*). This is a delicious summer dish which should be accompanied by new potatoes and fresh vegetables. If you don't have time to prepare the whole recipe, just sprinkle a skinned chicken breast with freshly ground black pepper, place under the grill for approximately 20 minutes and turn frequently to prevent burning. Serve with lots of fresh vegetables, new potatoes and a little gravy. Alternatively, choose one of the other dinner menus included in this diet.

As you perform the exercise programme today, be aware of just how much the fat-burner workout is actively helping you to burn away fat in readiness for your appearance on the beach in your swimsuit. Work out to some lively, strong-beat music performed by your favourite artist and really enjoy it. Have a great day.

DAY 2 FAT-BURNER FITNESS PROGRAMME

Mobilizing Warm-up

1. Shoulder rotations
Rotate both shoulders backwards
8 times, then forwards 8 times.

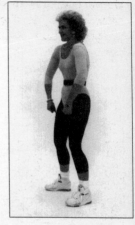

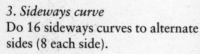

2. Alternate hip rotations
Rotate hips first in a clockwise
direction, then in an anti-
clockwise direction. Repeat 8
times (4 each direction).

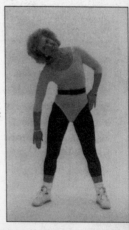

3. Sideways curve
Do 16 sideways curves to alternate
sides (8 each side).

4. *Waist twist*
With knees slightly bent and elbows bent outwards at shoulder level, twist upper body to alternate sides. Do 16 (8 each side).

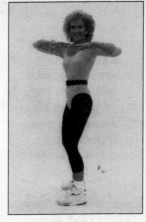

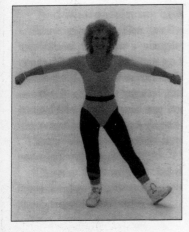

5. *Alternate heel digs to side*
Do 16 heel digs to alternate sides (8 each side), swinging arms out and in.

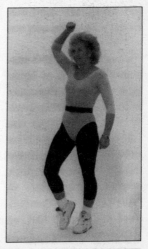

6. *Walking jog, arm circles*
As you step on the spot, circle alternate arms backwards. Do 12 circles (8 each arm).

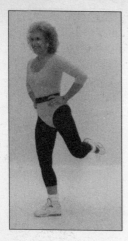

7. *Kick back*

Kick back alternate feet, bending the knee as you kick. Do 16 (8 each foot).

Stretches

8. *Calf stretch*

Stand with feet parallel, one foot in front of the other. Keeping the back leg straight and both heels on the floor, bend front knee as shown. Hold for 8 counts. Slowly release, and repeat with other leg in front.

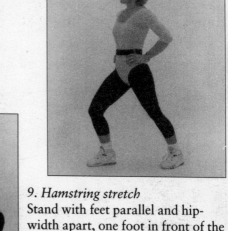

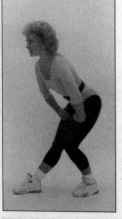

9. *Hamstring stretch*

Stand with feet parallel and hip-width apart, one foot in front of the other. Keep front leg straight and bend the knee of the other leg as shown, ensuring that both heels remain on the floor. Hold for 8 counts, then slowly release, and repeat with other leg in front.

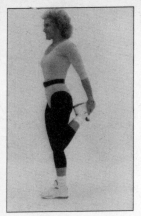

10. Front thigh stretch

Stand with feet together. Bend left leg and take hold of its foot with left hand as shown. Ease foot as close to seat as you can, and hold for 8 counts. Slowly release, and repeat with other leg.

11. Chest stretch

Stand with feet a comfortable distance apart. Extend arms behind you and, clasping the hands, raise arms as high as possible. Hold for 8 counts.

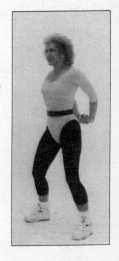

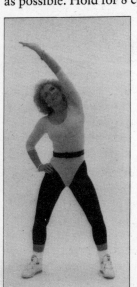

12. Waist stretch

Stand with feet a comfortable distance apart, one hand on hip. Reach other arm over to side with palm of hand facing ceiling. Hold for 10 counts. Slowly release, and repeat to other side.

Pulse-Raiser Warm-up

Follow exercises 13–22 at low-impact level.

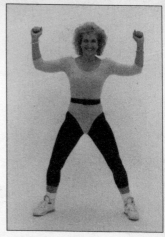

13. *Side steps*
Step from side to side, opening and closing bent arms as you step. Do 24 (12 each side).

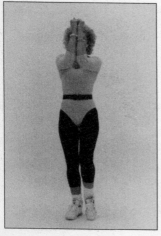

14. *Knee raises to opposite elbow*
Raise alternate knees towards opposite elbow. Do 16 (8 each knee).

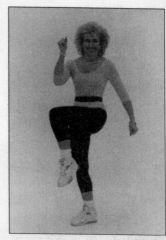

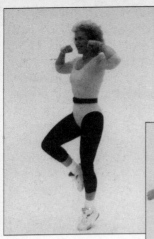

15. *Jogging, arm bends*
Jog on the spot, alternately bending and straightening arms out to sides at shoulder level. Do 24.

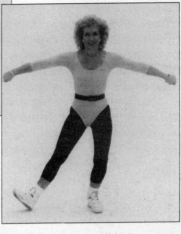

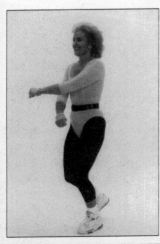

16. *Alternate heel digs to side*
Do 24 heel digs to alternate sides (12 each heel), swinging arms out to sides and then crossing them in front.

17. *Jogging, arms swinging*
Jog on the spot, swinging arms out to sides and then crossing them in front. Do 24.

18. Side steps

Step from side to side, swinging arms out to sides and then crossing them in front as you step.

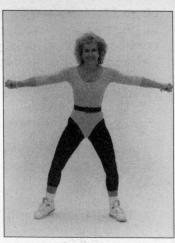

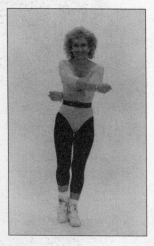

19. Forward and backward jogging

Stand with one leg in front of the other. Jog, transferring weight from one leg to the other, like a pendulum swinging. Do 16 with one leg in front, then change legs and repeat.

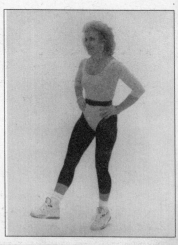

20. *Kick back and touch*
Kick back with alternate feet to touch opposite hand behind you and swinging other arm as high as you can. Repeat 16 times (8 each foot).

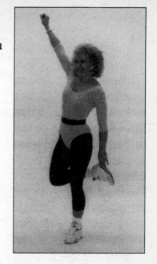

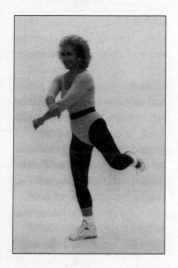

21. *Kick back*
Kick back with alternate feet, bending the knee as you kick and swinging arms out to sides and then crossing them in front. Do 24 (12 each foot).

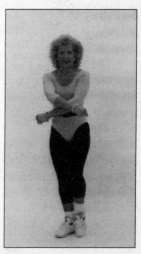

22. *Walking jog*
Walk on the spot, swinging arms out to sides and then crossing them in front. Do 24.

Fat-Burner Workout

Repeat exercises 13–22 at high-impact level (or low impact as necessary).

Cool Down

Repeat exercises 13–22 at low-impact level.

Repeat stretches 8–12.

DAY 2 DIET

Breakfast
12 oz (300 g) any fresh fruit, plus 5 oz (125 g) low-calorie, low-fat yogurt.

Lunch
Jacket potato (8 oz/200 g) topped with Carrot and Sultana Salad (*see recipe*), served with home-made Coleslaw (*see recipe*).

Dinner
Chicken with Orange and Apricots (*see recipe*), served with vegetables of your choice and 4 oz (100 g) new potatoes, followed by Raspberry Yogurt Delight (*see recipe*).

Two days of diet and exercise completed and you've suddenly discovered muscles in your body you didn't even know existed. But the good news is things are beginning to happen already. The fat stores are starting to diminish, the body is looking better and you should be feeling more energetic, despite the slight discomfort in some of your muscles. It would be my guess that the calf muscles are feeling a little sore today. This could be due to the fact that when you are performing your aerobic exercises you are not allowing your heels to touch the floor, but are remaining on the balls of your feet. The muscle soreness will lessen over the next two or three days, so just do whatever exercises you feel you can today, taking extra care to fully execute the stretches before and after the aerobic section. The reason for the delayed onset of muscle soreness is that your muscles have not been used to working so hard for some time and while the body has a built-in anaesthetic effect on muscles after exercising them for the first time, after about forty-eight hours this anaesthetic wears off and we feel the difference! If you continue exercising at a slightly gentler level today, by tomorrow your muscles should be feeling much more comfortable. Mild discomfort indicates that you have been working hard, and that is good, but if your muscles are seriously painful you must take it a lot easier.

If you are reading this prior to eating your breakfast, go and slip on your skirt or trousers and see if they feel any looser. If you have already eaten something today, then wait until tomorrow and try on either garment first thing when you get up.

I hope you enjoy today's crunchy breakfast, but don't eat any more than the 10 sultanas that have been allocated! Your fresh fruit lunch can include any type of fruit you wish – for instance, if you want to eat a whole pound of strawberries, go ahead. I also hope you enjoy the Ham, Beef and

Chicken Salad (*see recipe*). I always consider it a treat to be able to eat three meats at one time. If you don't have the variety to hand, or you don't have time to make this special salad, choose one of the other dinner menus instead. The Hot Cherries with Ice Cream (*see recipe*) is one of my favourite desserts. For a special occasion it can be made even more delicious by adding some cherry brandy to the juice. You should serve this dish immediately after pouring on the cherries as the ice cream will melt quickly.

Make sure you don't cheat today and best of luck with the exercises.

DAY 3 FAT-BURNER FITNESS PROGRAMME

Mobilizing Warm-up

1. Shoulder rotations
Rotate both shoulders
backwards 8 times, then
forwards 8 times.

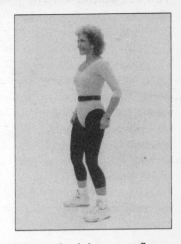

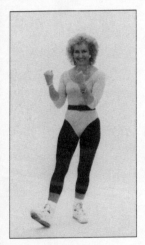

2. Alternate heel digs, arm flexes
Do 24 heel digs (12 each heel),
alternating heels and at the same
time flexing and straightening
the arms.

3. Alternate hip rotations
Rotate hips first in a
clockwise direction, then in
an anti-clockwise direction.
Do 8 alternate hip rotations
(4 each direction).

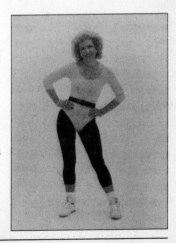

4. *Sideways curve*
Do 16 sideways curves to alternate sides (8 each side).

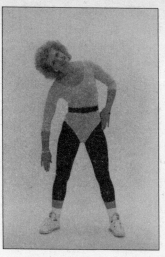

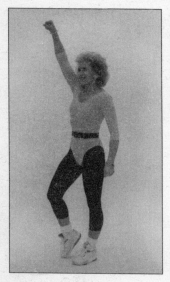

5. *Walking jog, arm circles*
Walk on the spot, circling one arm backwards 4 times. Repeat with other arm.

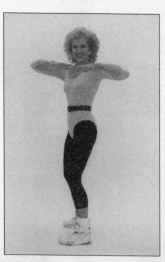

6. *Waist twist*
With knees slightly bent and elbows bent outwards at shoulder level, twist upper body to alternate sides. Do 8 (4 each side).

7. *Kick back*
With hands on hips, kick back
with alternate feet, bending the
knee as you kick. Do 24 (12 each
foot).

Stretches

8. *Hamstring stretch*
Stand with feet parallel and hip-
width apart, one foot in front of
the other. Keep front leg straight
and bend the knee of the other
leg as shown. Hold for 8 counts,
then slowly release, and repeat
with other leg in front.

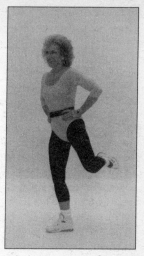

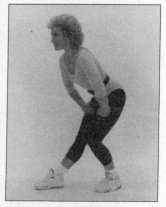

9. *Calf stretch*
Stand as shown with feet
parallel, one foot in front of the
other. Keeping both heels on the
floor, bend both knees and hold
for 8 counts. Slowly release, and
repeat with other leg in front.

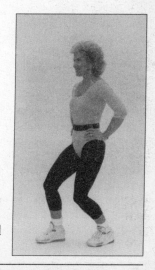

10. Front thigh stretch

Stand with feet together. Bend left leg and take hold of its foot with left hand as shown. Ease foot as close to seat as you can, and hold for 8 counts. Slowly release, and repeat with other leg.

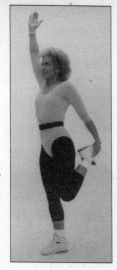

11. Tricep stretch

Stand with feet a comfortable distance apart and knees slightly bent. Ease one arm across chest, holding it above the elbow with the other hand. Hold for 8 seconds. Slowly release, and repeat with the other arm.

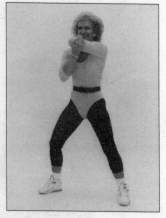

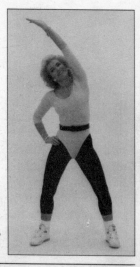

12. Waist stretch

Stand with feet a comfortable distance apart and one hand on hip. Reach other arm over to side with palm of hand facing ceiling. Hold for 8 counts. Slowly release, and repeat to other side.

13. Upper back stretch

Stand with feet a comfortable distance apart, knees slightly bent. Extend both arms in front of you and clasp hands together. Hold for 8 counts.

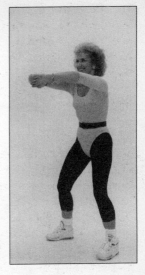

Pulse-Raiser Warm-up

Follow exercises 14–23 at low-impact level.

14. Step and kick

Step with one foot and then kick across with other foot, swinging both arms to opposite side as you kick. Do 24 to alternate sides (12 each foot).

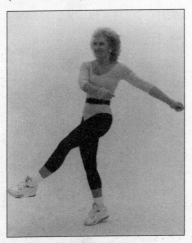

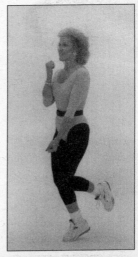

15. Jogging, arms flexing

Jog on the spot, flexing alternate arms as you go. Do 24.

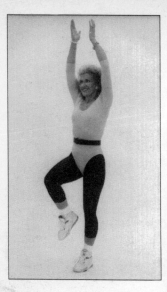

16. *March and clap*

March on the spot, clapping hands above head. Do 24.

17. *Knee raises to opposite elbow*

Raise alternate knees towards opposite elbow. Do 16 raises (8 each knee).

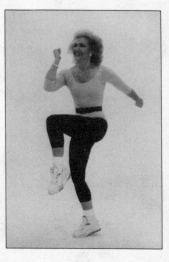

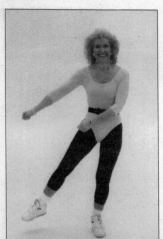

18. *Sideways jogging*

Jog from side to side, swinging arms as you go. Do 16 (8 each side).

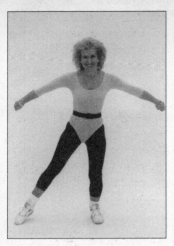

19. *Step and point*
Extend one leg out to the side and point that foot, swinging arms out to sides. Bring leg and arms back in again, and repeat to other side. Do 16 to alternate sides (8 each side).

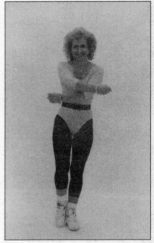

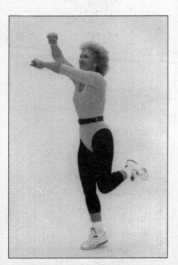

20. *Kick back, arms high*
Kick back with alternate feet, raising arms and swinging them out and across. Do 16 (8 each foot).

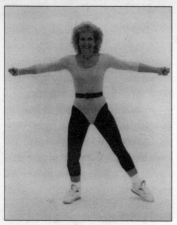

21. *Step and point*
Extend one leg out to the side and point that foot, swinging arms out to sides. Bring leg and arms back in again, and repeat to other side. Do 16 to alternate sides (8 each side).

22. *Jogging, arms bending*
Jog on the spot, bending arms out and in at shoulder level. Do 16.

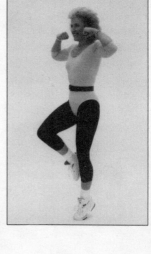

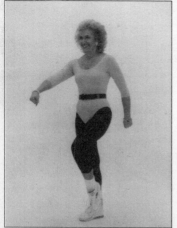

23. Marching
March on the spot, swinging arms as you go. Do 32 steps.

Fat-Burner Workout

Repeat exercises 14–23 at high-impact level (or low-impact as necessary).

Cool Down

Repeat exercises 14, 15, 19, 21 and 23 at low-impact level.

Repeat stretches 8–13.

<u>DAY 3 DIET</u>

Breakfast
5 oz (125 g) natural yogurt mixed with 1 tablespoon branflakes, 1 teaspoon honey and 10 sultanas.

Lunch
16 oz (400 g) any fresh fruit, plus 1 diet yogurt.

Dinner
Ham, Beef and Chicken salad (*see recipe*), then Hot Cherries and Ice Cream (*see recipe*).

You are now halfway through the first week of the 14-day programme. Hopefully the garment that was so tight on Day 1 is now significantly looser and your muscles have come to terms with the increased physical activity which has become part of your everyday life. In your workout today try to be as energetic as possible, recognizing that the fat-burner workout is actively helping you to lose that unwanted flab in readiness for your holiday. Not only does aerobic exercise help to burn away fat, but it also increases the flow of oxygen to the skin, thus enabling it to shrink as you lose weight and inches, and stay firm. As well as working your heart and lungs, exercise is one of the best beauty treatments you can possibly have.

I hope you are enjoying the diet. The Spinach and Mushroom Salad (*see recipe*) which is suggested for today's lunch is brimming with vitamins and constitutes the ideal meal for health and vitality. If fresh spinach is difficult to find, then make up your own salad according to what you have available. Really pile up the plate with tomatoes, lettuce, cucumber, watercress, peppers – they are all so low in calories that we can eat loads of them without any detriment to our waistline.

One of the best ways to prevent overeating during our evening meal is to have a couple of glasses of diet drink beforehand. These will have the effect of filling your tummy and taking the edge off your appetite. The problem with having to wait some considerable time for the evening meal is that we become so hungry that we eat a significant amount before it actually has time to reach the stomach itself. Consequently, we keep on eating because we still feel hungry, and then all of a sudden the food arrives in the stomach and we feel overfull. This is just what we don't want when we're trying to lose weight for our holiday. I regularly drink a couple of cans of caffeine-free diet coke prior to my evening meal and it really helps me to regulate the quantities that I eat.

The Summer Lamb Stew (*see recipe*) is very satisfying and combined with lots of fresh green vegetables is an ideal way to fill up if you're feeling peckish. The Melon with Strawberries (*see recipe*) brings the meal to a delicious conclusion.

Now that you are halfway through your week it is a good idea to get going on your holiday preparations. Start by making a list of outstanding items that you need to buy for the holiday (see **Planning Your Packing** on page 188 for some ideas). Also, make a list of those people to whom you will be sending postcards and ensure that you have their correct addresses. Write the addresses in your diary or on a piece of paper that can be safely stored away in your suitcase. It's these finer details that often get forgotten as panic sets in nearer to departure date.

DAY 4 FAT-BURNER FITNESS PROGRAMME

Mobilizing Warm-up

1. Shoulder rotations
Rotate alternate shoulders backwards 8 times, then forwards 8 times (4 each shoulder). Then repeat, rotating both shoulders together.

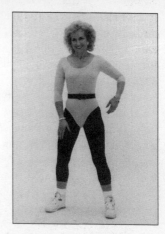

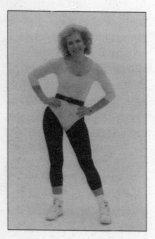

2. Alternate hip rotations
Rotate hips first in a clockwise direction, then in an anti-clockwise direction. Repeat alternate hip rotations 8 times (4 each direction).

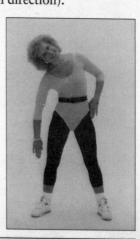

3. Sideways curve
Do 16 sideways curves to alternate sides (8 each side).

4. Alternate heel digs, arm swings

Do 24 heel digs (12 each heel), alternating heels and swinging arms out to sides and then crossing them in front.

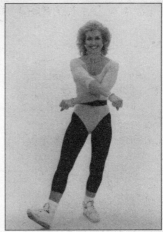

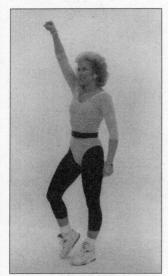

5. Walking jog, arm circles

Walk on the spot and circle one arm forwards 4 times. Repeat with other arm. Repeat, circling arms backwards.

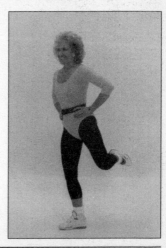

6. Kick Back

With hands on hips, kick back with alternate feet, bending the knee as you kick. Do 16 (8 each foot).

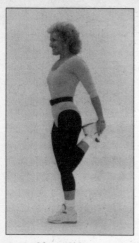

Stretches

7. *Front thigh stretch*
Stand with feet together. Bend left leg and take hold of its foot with left hand as shown. Ease foot as close to seat as you can and hold for 8 counts. Slowly release, and repeat with other leg.

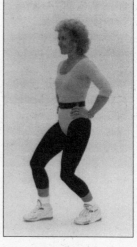

8. *Calf stretch*
Stand as shown with feet parallel, one foot in front of the other. Keeping both heels on the floor, bend both knees and hold for 8 counts. Slowly release, and repeat with other leg in front.

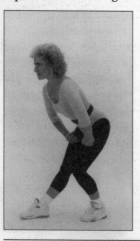

9. *Hamstring stretch*
Stand with feet parallel and hip-width apart, one foot in front of the other. Keep front leg straight and bend the knee of the other leg as shown ensuring that both heels remain on the floor. Hold for 8 counts, slowly release, and repeat with other leg in front.

10. Chest stretch
Stand with feet a comfortable distance apart. Extend arms behind you and, clasping the hands, raise arms as high as possible. Hold for 8 counts.

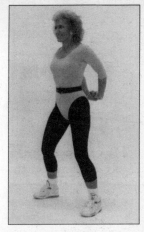

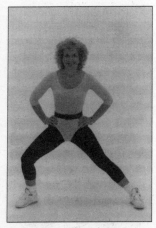

11. Inner thigh stretch
Stand with feet wide apart with one foot turned out to the side slightly and the knee bent directly over that foot. Keep the other leg straight, with foot parallel, and hold for 8 counts. Slowly release, change legs and repeat.

Pulse-Raiser Warm-up

Follow exercises 12–22 at low-impact level.

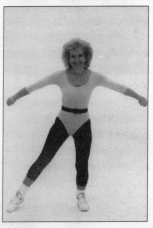

12. Step and point
Extend one leg out to the side, pointing the foot, and at the same time swing arms out to sides. Bring leg and arms in again, and repeat to the other side. Do 16 (8 each side).

13. Sideways jogging
Jog from side to side,
swinging arms as you go.
Do 16.

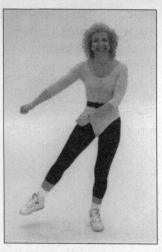

14. Kick back and touch
Kick back with alternate
feet to touch opposite hand
behind you and swinging
other arm as high as you
can. Do 16 (8 each foot)

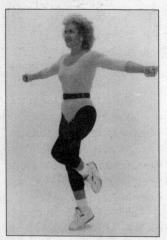

15. Jogging, arms swinging
Jog on the spot, swinging
arms out to sides and then
crossing them in front.
Do 24.

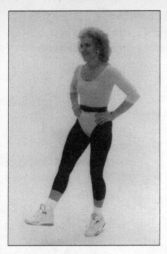

16. *Forward and backward jogging*
Stand with one leg in front of the other. Jog, transferring weight from one leg to the other, like a pendulum swinging. Do 16 with one leg in front, then change legs and repeat.

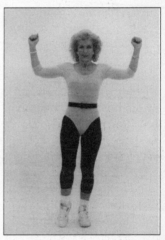

17. *Walking jog, arms in and out*
Walk on the spot, swinging bent arms in and out at shoulder level. Do 16.

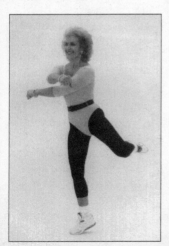

18. *Kick back*
Kick back with alternate feet, bending the knee as you kick and, at the same time, swinging arms out to sides and then crossing them in front. Do 16 (8 each foot).

19. Arm swinging
Swing arms from side to side, bending the knees and transferring weight from one foot to the other as you go. Do 16 (8 each side).

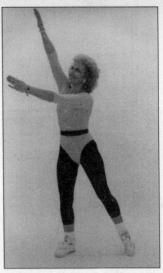

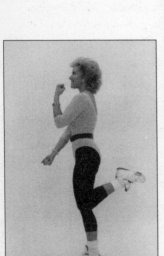

20. Jogging
Jog on the spot, kicking feet high behind you and flexing alternate arms in front. Do 16 (8 each foot).

21. Alternate knee raises
Raise alternate knees, bringing bent arms out to sides and in at shoulder level. Do 16 (8 each knee).

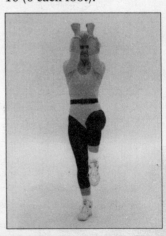

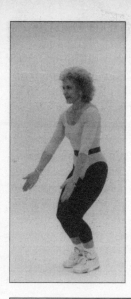

22. *Ski down*
Stand with feet together, arms upstretched. Bend knees and swing arms down to your sides. Return to start and repeat, swinging arms up and down. Do 16.

Fat-Burner Workout
Repeat exercises 12–21 at high-impact level (or low-impact as necessary).

Cool Down
Repeat exercises 12–22 at low-impact level.

Repeat stretches 7–11.

DAY 4 DIET

Breakfast
1 oz (25 g) toast, plus 8 oz (200 g) tin baked beans.

Lunch
Spinach and Mushroom Salad (*see recipe*).

or

Large mixed salad with 3 oz (75 g) chicken or lean ham, plus 1 tablespoon Reduced-Oil Salad Dressing (*see recipe*) and 1/2 oz (12.5 g) bread.

Dinner
Summer Lamb Stew (*see recipe*) with green vegetables as desired, and Melon with Strawberries (*see recipe*).

Let today's first task be trying on the skirt or trousers to see how much looser they have become. I hope your body has recovered from the earlier exercises and is now feeling fitter by the day. Try to increase the level of activity during your workout and feel the energy beginning to generate. Today, pay attention to your posture and pull your tummy in whenever you think of it. Also, try to remember to keep your shoulders back and make your posture more upright. Endeavour to be more energetic in all that you do whether at home or at work. Use the stairs rather than the lift and perhaps walk rather than taking the car for every journey. You should now be feeling significantly slimmer and fitter and maybe there is a spring in your step now that you know you are winning.

Take another look at the holiday brochures and read through all the details of the hotel or apartment where you plan to stay. Imagine the sunshine, imagine the feeling of freedom and relaxation and imagine how good you're going to feel because you've lost weight and inches (cm).

As your newsagent will probably want seven days' notice, now is the time to cancel any newspapers or magazines that may be due for delivery during your absence. If you need a repeat prescription for any medication, now is the time to order it. Are there any toiletries that you require for the holiday and what about films for the camera? Check these against your 'packing check list'. Have you received your air tickets and have you checked that all the details are correct? Is your passport still valid and what about the rest of the family's? Check these things now while you have time to make any adjustments or renewals. Have you ordered your travellers' cheques and currency? Make a list of the jobs that you need to do and tick them off one by one as you complete them. There is no better feeling than going on holiday when you have been thoroughly organized and everything is under control.

Today's menus include a high-fibre breakfast, ham and salad sandwiches and fruit for lunch, and Fish Cakes (*see recipe*) for dinner. You could serve your fish cakes either with tomato ketchup or a low-fat parsley sauce made with skimmed milk from the daily allowance, plus cornflour, chopped onion, plenty of seasoning and chopped parsley. You don't need too many potatoes because there is potato in the fish cakes themselves, but fill up on lots of fresh vegetables such as carrots, broccoli and mange-tout. The Gooseberry Fool (*see recipe*) is a delightful dessert, but if you don't have time for the preparation, stick to a simple fruit salad topped with a little low-fat yogurt.

Enjoy your workout and congratulate yourself on the fact that you're nearly at the end of the first week. Don't cheat – I promise it will be worth it in the end.

DAY 5 FAT-BURNER FITNESS PROGRAMME

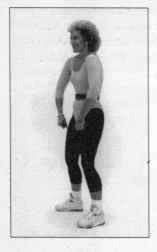

Mobilizing Warm-up

1. Shoulder rotations
Rotate both shoulders
backwards 8 times, then
forwards 8 times.

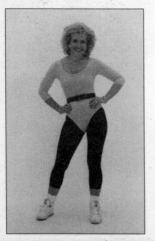

2. Walking jog
Walk on the spot, swinging
arms as you step. Do 16 steps.

3. Alternate hip rotations
Rotate hips first in a clockwise
direction, then in an anti-
clockwise direction. Repeat
alternate hip rotations 8 times
(4 each direction).

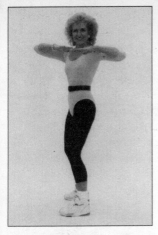

4. Waist twist
With knees slightly bent and elbows bent outwards at shoulder level, twist upper body to alternate sides. Do 16 to alternate sides (8 each side).

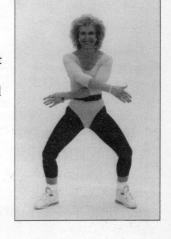

5. Arm circles
Standing with feet wide apart and knees bent, swing both arms out and around in a full circle, crossing them in front of you. Do 4 inward circles and 4 outward circles.

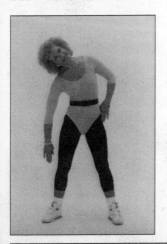

6. Sideways curve
Do 16 sideways curves to alternate sides (8 each side).

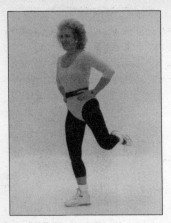

7. *Kick back*
With hands on hips, kick back with alternate feet, bending the knee as you kick. Do 16 (8 each foot).

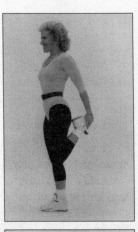

Stretches

8. *Front thigh stretch*
Stand with feet together. Bend left leg and take hold of its foot with left hand as shown. Ease foot as close to seat as you can and hold for 8 counts. Slowly release, and repeat with other leg.

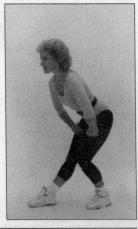

9. *Hamstring stretch*
Stand with feet parallel and hip-width apart, one foot in front of the other. Keep front leg straight and bend the knee of the other leg as shown ensuring that both heels remain on the floor. Hold for 8 counts. Raise the toes of the straight leg and hold for a further 8 counts. Slowly release, and repeat with other leg in front.

10. Tricep stretch

Stand with feet a comfortable distance apart and knees slightly bent. Ease one arm across chest holding it above the elbow with the other hand. Hold for 8 seconds. Slowly release, and repeat with other arm.

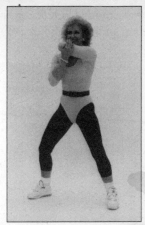

11. Inner thigh and upper back stretch

Stand with feet wide apart with one foot turned out to the side slightly and the knee bent directly over that foot. Keep the other leg straight, with foot parallel. Extend both arms in front at shoulder level and clasp hands with palms facing outwards. Hold for 8 counts. Slowly straighten leg, then repeat to other side.

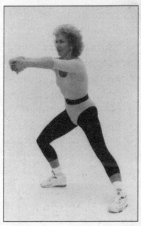

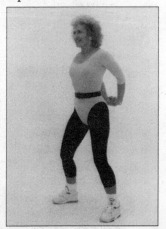

12. Chest stretch

Stand with feet a comfortable distance apart. Extend arms behind you and, clasping the hands, raise arms as high as possible. Hold for 8 counts.

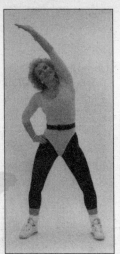

13. *Waist stretch*

Stand with feet a comfortable distance apart. Reach one arm over to side with palm of hand facing ceiling. Hold for 8 counts. Slowly release, and repeat to other side.

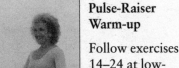

Pulse-Raiser Warm-up

Follow exercises 14–24 at low-impact level.

14. *Knee raises*

Raise alternate knees and at the same time draw hands forward and back, as if opening and closing a drawer. Do 24 raises (12 each knee).

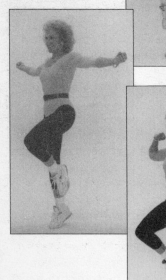

15. *Jogging, arm bends*

Jog on the spot, alternately bending and straightening arms out to sides at shoulder level. Do 24 steps.

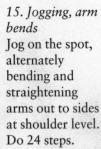

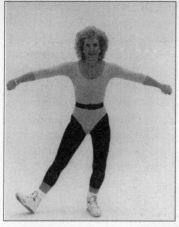

16. Alternate heel digs to side
Do 24 heel digs to alternate sides (12 each side), swinging arms out to sides and crossing them in front.

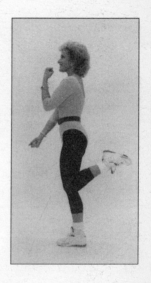

17. Jogging
Jog on the spot, kicking feet high behind you and flexing alternate arms in front. Do 24 (12 each foot).

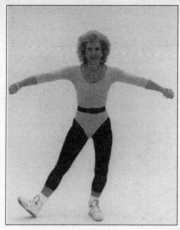

18. Marching, arms out and in
March on the spot, swinging arms out to sides and then crossing them in front. Do 24 steps.

19. *Kick back*
Kick back with alternate feet, bending the knee as you kick and, at the same time, swinging arms out to sides and then crossing them in front. Do 16 (8 each foot).

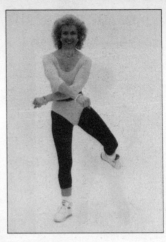

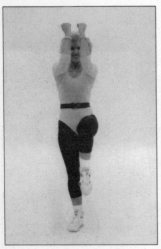

20. *Knee raises, arms out and in*
Raise alternate knees, bringing bent arms out and in at shoulder level. Do 16 knee raises (8 each knee).

21. *Forward and backward jogging*
Stand with one leg in front of the other. Jog, transferring weight from one leg to the other, like a pendulum swinging. Do 16 with one leg in front, then change legs and repeat.

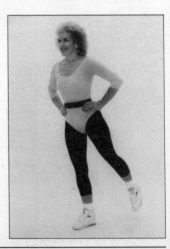

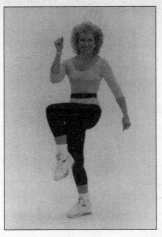

22. *Knee raises to opposite elbow*
Raise alternate knees towards opposite elbow. Do 16 (8 each knee).

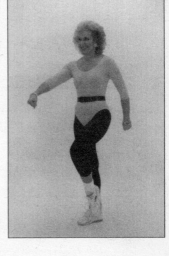

23. *Marching*
March on the spot. Do 32 steps.

24. *Ski down*
Stand with feet together, arms upstretched. Bend knees and swing arms down. Return to start and repeat, swinging arms up and down. Do 18.

Fat-Burner Workout

Repeat exercises 15–22 at high-impact level (or low-impact as necessary).

Cool Down

Repeat exercises 15–24 at low-impact level.

Repeat stretches 8–13.

DAY 5 DIET

Breakfast
1¹/2 oz (37.5 g) Fruit and Fibre, plus milk from allowance and 1 teaspoon sugar.

Lunch
2 slices (2 oz/50 g) bread spread with Reduced-Oil Salad Dressing (*see recipe*) and mustard, and filled with 1 oz (25 g) ham and salad, plus 1 piece fresh fruit.

Dinner
Fish Cakes (*see recipe*) served with unlimited vegetables, followed by Gooseberry Fool (*see recipe*).

Tomorrow is weighing and measuring day. Today, try to be extra strict and really energetic during your workout. Try not to eat your evening meal too late so that it can be properly digested before you go to bed. Also, try and be as active throughout the day as you can. If you have a fitness video, make the time to work out to that too. Alternatively, play a game of sport or attend an aerobics class. Make a real effort to give your metabolism a boost so that the scales and tape measure will have 'glad tidings' for you in the morning.

Spend some time planning your outfits for the holiday and make a list of outstanding items of clothing that you require. Check that any arrangements made to look after your pets are in order and that you have asked someone to water your plants while you are away.

Security when going on holiday is always a problem and there are some useful tips on page 191 to help prevent unwelcome visitors. It is also a good idea to ask a responsible neighbour or friend to visit your house on a regular basis to check that all is well.

Keep yourself really busy and don't even think about cheating. You are so close to the end of your first week that it is absolutely essential you are self-disciplined today. Best of luck tomorrow morning.

DAY 6 FAT-BURNER FITNESS PROGRAMME

Mobilizing Warm-up

1. Shoulder rotations
Rotate alternate shoulders backwards 8 times, then forwards 8 times (4 each shoulder). Then repeat, rotating both shoulders together.

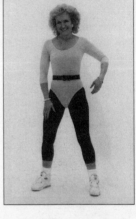

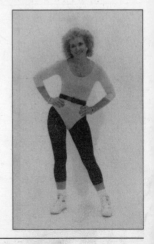

2. Alternate heel digs, arm flexes
Do 24 heel digs (12 each heel), alternating heels and at the same time flexing and straightening the arms.

3. Alternate hip rotations
Rotate hips first in a clockwise direction, then in an anti-clockwise direction. Repeat alternate hip rotations 8 times (4 each direction).

4. *Sideways curve*
Do 16 sideways curves to alternate sides (8 each side).

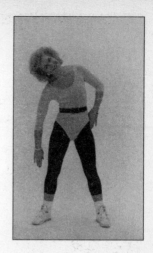

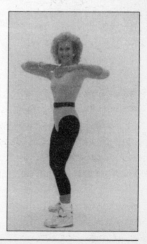

5. *Walking jog, arm circles*
Walk on the spot and circle one arm backwards 4 times. Repeat with other arm. Repeat, circling arms forwards.

6. *Waist twist*
With knees slightly bent and elbows bent outwards at shoulder level, twist upper body to alternate sides. Do 16 to alternate sides (8 each side).

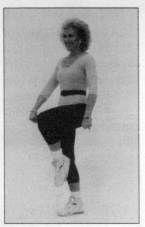

7. *Knee raises*
Raise alternate knees and at the same time draw hands forward and back, as if opening and closing a drawer. Do 24 raises (12 each knee).

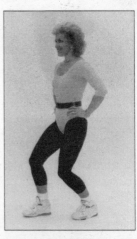

Stretches

8. *Calf stretch*
Stand as shown with feet parallel, one foot in front of the other. Keeping both heels on the floor, bend both knees and hold for 8 counts. Slowly release, and repeat with other leg in front.

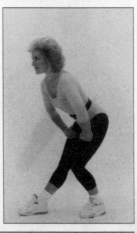

9. *Hamstring stretch*
Stand with feet parallel and hip-width apart, one foot in front of the other. Keep front leg straight and bend the knee of the other leg as shown ensuring that both heels remain on the floor. Hold for 8 counts. Raise the toes of the straight leg and hold for a further 8 counts. Slowly release, and repeat with other leg in front.

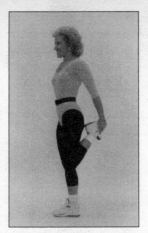

10. *Front thigh stretch*
Stand with feet together. Bend left leg and take hold of its foot with left hand as shown. Ease foot as close to seat as you can and hold for 8 counts. Slowly release, and repeat with other leg.

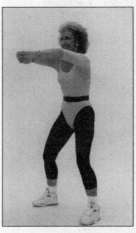

11. *Upper back stretch*
Stand with feet a comfortable distance apart, knees slightly bent. Extend both arms in front of you and clasp hands together. Hold for 8 counts.

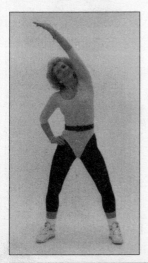

12. *Waist stretch*
Stand with feet a comfortable distance apart. Reach one arm over to side with palm of hand facing ceiling. Hold for 8 counts. Slowly release, and repeat to other side.

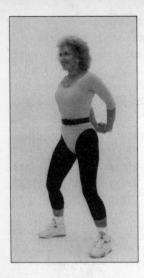

13. *Chest stretch*
Stand with feet a comfortable distance apart. Extend arms behind you and, clasping the hands, raise arms as high as possible. Hold for 8 counts.

Pulse-Raiser Warm-up

Follow exercises 14–24 at low-impact level.

14. *Alternate heel digs to side*
Do 24 heel digs to alternate sides (12 each side), swinging arms out to sides and crossing them in front.

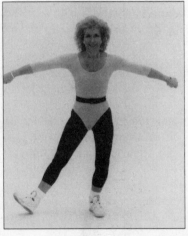

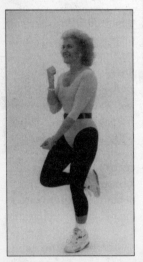

15. *Jogging, arms flexing*
Jog on the spot, flexing alternate arms. Do 16.

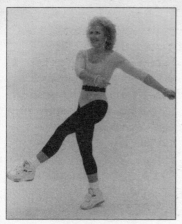

16. *Step and kick*
Step with one foot and kick across with the other foot, swinging arms to opposite side. Do 16 to alternate sides (8 each side).

17. *Walking jog, arms in and out*
Walk on the spot, swinging bent arms in and out at shoulder level. Do 16.

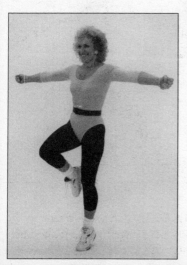

18. *Jogging, arm bends*
Jog on the spot, alternately bending and straightening arms out to sides at shoulder level. Do 24 steps.

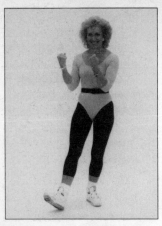

19. *Alternate heel digs, arm flexes*
Do 16 heel digs (8 each heel), alternating heels and at the same time flexing and straightening the arms.

20. *Jogging, arms swinging*
Jog on the spot, swinging arms out to sides and then crossing them in front as you go. Do 16.

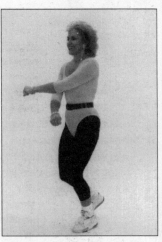

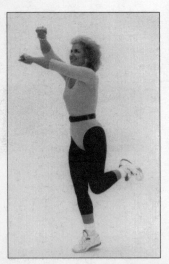

21. *Jogging, arms raising*
Continue jogging, but this time raise and lower arms as they swing and cross. Do 16.

22. *Knee raises to opposite elbow*
Raise alternate knees towards opposite elbow. Do 16 (8 each knee).

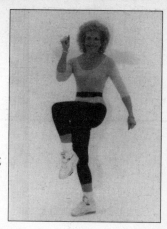

23. *Forward and backward jogging*
Stand with one leg in front of the other. Jog, transferring weight from one leg to the other, like a pendulum swinging. Do 16 with one leg in front, then change legs and repeat.

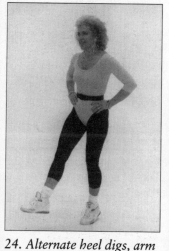

24. *Alternate heel digs, arm flexes*
Do 24 heel digs (12 each heel), alternating heels and at the same time flexing and straightening the arms.

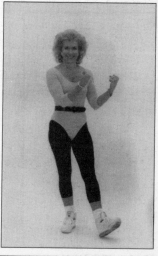

Fat-Burner Workout

Repeat exercises 14–24 twice at high-impact level (or low-impact as necessary).

Cool Down

Repeat exercises 14–24 at low-impact level.

Repeat stretches 8–13.

DAY 6 DIET

Breakfast
1 banana (any size) chopped into 2 x 5 oz (125 g) cartons raspberry-flavoured, low-calorie, low-fat yogurt.

Lunch
Mixed salad with 4 oz (100 g) jacket potato, topped with cottage cheese mixed with 2 oz (50 g) sweetcorn, plus 1 tablespoon Reduced-Oil Salad Dressing (*see recipe*).

Dinner
Glazed Chicken (*see recipe*) served with vegetables of your choice and 4 oz (100 g) boiled new potatoes, plus Summer Pots (*see recipe*).

Congratulations on reaching your first weighing and measuring day. You have been on the diet for six whole days and there should be a significant change in both your weight and your measurements. Make sure you weigh and measure yourself before you eat or drink anything today and carefully note the details on the **Measurement Record Chart** on page 16. Now that you have stuck to the diet and exercise programme for six days and are able to enjoy some of the benefits of feeling and looking slimmer, you will be all fired up to carry on for the remaining eight days. I have suggested that you weigh yourself today rather than tomorrow for one very good reason. Generally speaking we lose more weight in the first week of dieting, therefore I'm giving you the benefit of an extra day during the second week for you to make real progress so that you will see a substantial difference on the scales before you go on holiday. You are almost halfway through the 14-day campaign and since the first part is always the most difficult, you are now well on the way to success and a slimmer you to take on holiday.

You must be coping with the exercises a lot more easily now, even though the activity is stepped up and you are repeating the peak aerobic section at high- and low-impact level three times. This will very effectively increase the amount of fat that you burn away and will make you feel significantly fitter by the time you depart on holiday next week. Be as energetic as you possibly can throughout the day, always taking the physical option of walking rather than riding whenever possible.

Next week will be busy as you continue to plan your holiday wardrobe, trimming down the amount of luggage that you will take and yet packing sufficient clothes to give you lots of variety and different looks. Today would be a good day for writing out your luggage labels so that it is one task already completed. Also, start thinking about jewellery and accessories to complement your various outfits. Different-coloured belts and scarves take up very little space in a suitcase, but can dress up or down an outfit to make it look dramatically different from one day to another. Hair accessories can be a real boon on holiday when our hair needs to be dressed up after constant swimming. Brightly coloured butterfly clips and combs can give us a very sophisticated look.

Try to be really strict on the diet again today – no eating between meals. Remember the trick of drinking a low-calorie drink prior to meal times. In this final week we need all the help we can get to stay on course.

If you fancy something more exciting than toast and marmalade for breakfast, then choose from one of the other breakfast options. The Chicken or Prawn Chop Suey (*see recipe*) makes a delicious dinner and is very easy to prepare.

Only seven more days to go, so be good and look forward to being quite a lot slimmer by this time next week.

DAY 7 FAT-BURNER FITNESS PROGRAMME

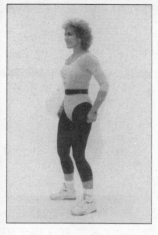

Mobilizing Warm-up

1. Shoulder rotations
Rotate both shoulders backwards 8 times, then forwards 8 times.

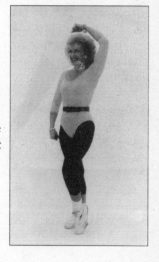

2. Walking jog, arm circles
Walk on the spot and circle one arm backwards 8 times. Repeat with other arm.

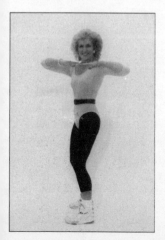

3. Waist twist
With knees slightly bent and elbows bent outwards at shoulder level, twist upper body to alternate sides. Do 16 to alternate sides (8 each side).

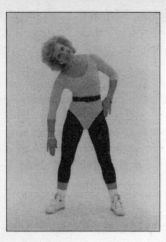

4. Sideways curve
Do 16 sideways curves to alternate sides (8 each side).

5. Knee raises
Raise alternate knees and at the same time draw hands forward and back, as if opening and closing a drawer. Do 16 raises (8 each knee).

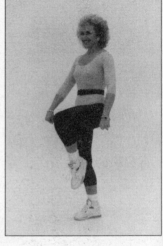

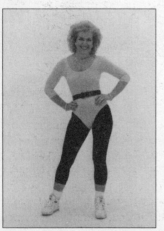

6. Alternate hip rotations
Rotate hips first in a clockwise direction, then in an anti-clockwise direction. Repeat alternate hip rotations 8 times (4 each direction).

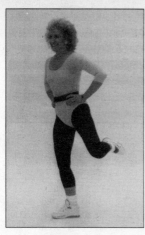

7. *Kick back*
Kick back with alternate feet, bending the knee as you kick. Do 16 (8 each foot).

Stretches

8. *Calf stretch*
Stand as shown (below right) with feet parallel, one foot in front of the other. Keeping both heels on the floor, bend both knees and hold for 8 counts. Slowly release, and repeat with other leg in front.

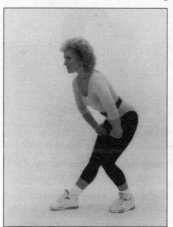

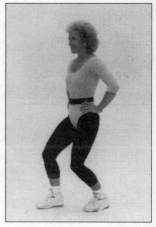

9. *Hamstring stretch*
Stand with feet parallel and hip-width apart, one foot in front of the other. Keep front leg straight and bend the knee of the other leg as shown ensuring that both heels remain on the floor. Hold for 8 counts. Raise the toes of the straight leg and hold for a further 8 counts. Slowly release, and repeat with other leg in front.

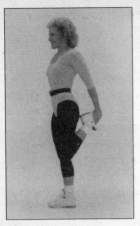

10. *Front thigh stretch*
Stand with feet together. Bend left leg and take hold of its foot with left hand as shown. Ease foot as close to seat as you can and hold for 8 counts. Slowly release, and repeat with other leg.

11. *Waist stretch*
Stand with feet a comfortable distance apart. Reach one arm over to side with palm of hand facing ceiling. Hold for 8 counts. Slowly release, and repeat to other side.

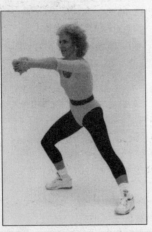

12. *Inner thigh and upper back stretch*
Stand with feet wide apart with one foot turned out to the side slightly and the knee bent directly over that foot. Keep the other leg straight, with foot parallel. Extend both arms in front at shoulder level and clasp hands with palms facing outwards. Hold for 8 counts. Slowly straighten leg, then repeat to other side.

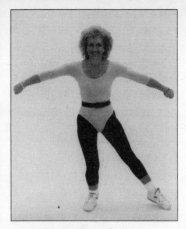

Pulse-Raiser Warm-up

Follow exercises 13–22 at low-impact level.

13. *Step and point*
Extend one leg out to the side, pointing the foot, and at the same time swing arms out to sides. Bring leg and arms in again, crossing arms in front, then repeat to the other side. Do 16 (8 each side).

14. *Kick back and touch*
Kick back with alternate feet to touch opposite hand behind you and swinging other arm as high as you can. Repeat 16 times (8 each foot).

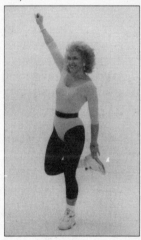

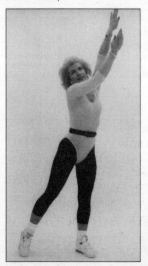

15. *Arm swinging*
Swing arms from side to side, bending the knees and transferring weight from one foot to the other as you go. Make big sweeping movements. Do 8 (4 each side).

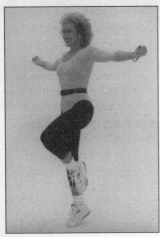

16. Knee raises, arms out and in
Raise alternate knees, bringing bent arms out and in at shoulder level. Do 16 knee raises (8 each knee).

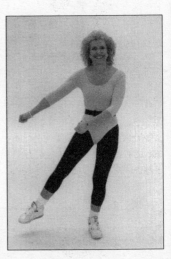

17. Sideways jogging
Jog from side to side, swinging arms as you go. Do 16.

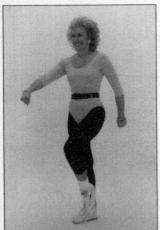

18. Marching
March on the spot. Do 16 steps.

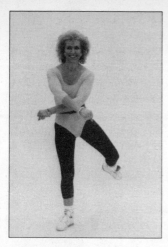

19. Kick back
Kick back with alternate feet, bending the knee as you kick and, at the same time, swinging arms out to sides and then crossing them in front. Do 16 (8 each foot).

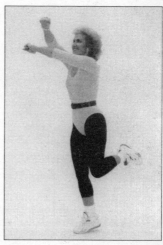

20. Kick back
Continue to kick back with alternate feet, raising arms as you swing them out and across. Do 16 (8 each foot).

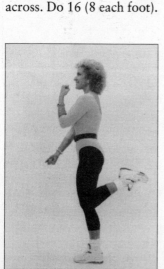

21. Jogging
Jog on the spot, kicking feet high behind you and flexing alternate arms in front. Do 16 (8 each foot).

22. *Walking jog*
Do a walking jog, swinging arms out to sides and then crossing them in front as you jog. Do 24.

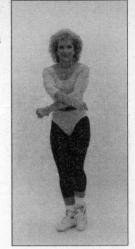

Fat-Burner Workout

Repeat exercises 13–22 at high-impact level (or low-impact as necessary).

Cool Down

Repeat exercises 13–22 at low-impact level.

Repeat stretches 8–12.

DAY 7 DIET

Breakfast
1¹/₂ oz (37.5 g) toast spread with 3 teaspoons marmalade.

Lunch
1 slimmers' cup-a-soup, plus 1 roll filled with 2 oz (50 g) salmon and cucumber mixed with Reduced-Oil Salad Dressing (*see recipe*), plus salad vegetables.

Dinner
Chicken or Prawn Chop Suey (*see recipe*) with 4 oz (100 g) boiled brown rice (dry weight), followed by Melon Sundae (*see recipe*).

It's time to try on the skirt (or trousers) again. I do hope it is much looser than it was a week ago. You are now on the countdown to your holiday so there will be lots to do and plenty of jobs to keep your mind off food. If you haven't got time to prepare the recipes as suggested, remember you can always have a straightforward grilled piece of chicken or microwaved white fish instead, served with lots of vegetables. Dessert can be as simple as a yogurt and a piece of fruit. Remind yourself of the dinner and dessert options available to you by referring to the menus in the **Free Choice Diet** chapter. I hope you enjoy the jacket potato with baked beans for your lunch. This is a firm favourite of mine as I always feel I've had a substantial meal afterwards. This evening's meal is something of a celebration after completing eight days of dieting. Enjoy it.

Have you started preparing your small bottles of cosmetics so that you save as much valuable space as possible in your suitcase? See **Planning Your Packing** for further tips. It's a good idea to get these time-consuming but worthwhile chores out of the way. If you have access to a photocopier it is advisable to make two photocopies of your credit cards, driving licence, passport and travel tickets, just in case they get mislaid or stolen. Keep one copy of each at home and put the other in a sealed envelope away from the original documents. Storing it in your suitcase is probably the best bet.

Work out today with extra energy and enthusiasm and keep reminding yourself that the effort put in now will make you look so much better in your swimsuit in a week's time.

DAY 8 FAT-BURNER FITNESS PROGRAMME

Mobilizing Warm-up

1. Shoulder rotations
Rotate both shoulders backwards 8
times, then forwards 8 times.

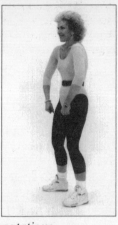

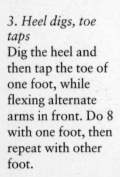

2. Alternate hip rotations
Rotate hips first in a clockwise
direction, then in an anti-clockwise
direction. Repeat alternate hip
rotations 8 times (4 each direction).

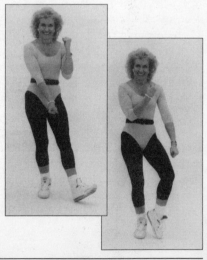

*3. Heel digs, toe
taps*
Dig the heel and
then tap the toe of
one foot, while
flexing alternate
arms in front. Do 8
with one foot, then
repeat with other
foot.

4. *Walking jog, arm circles*

Do a walking jog on the spot, circling alternate arms backwards as you step. Do 16 circles (8 each arm).

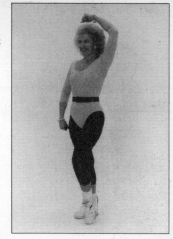

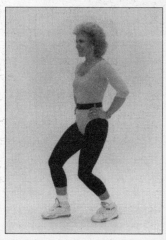

5. *Waist twist*

With knees slightly bent and elbows bent outwards at shoulder level, twist upper body to alternate sides. Do 16 to alternate sides (8 each side).

Stretches

6. *Calf stretch*

Stand as shown with feet parallel, one foot in front of the other. Keeping both heels on the floor, bend both knees and hold for 8 counts. Slowly release, and repeat with other leg in front.

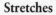

7. *Hamstring stretch*

Stand with feet parallel and hip-width apart, one foot in front of the other. Keep front leg straight and bend the knee of the other leg as shown ensuring that both heels remain on the floor. Hold for 8 counts. Raise the toes of the straight leg and hold for a further 8 counts. Slowly release, and repeat with other leg in front.

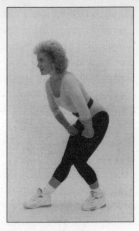

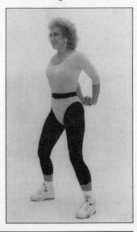

8. *Front thigh stretch*

Stand with feet together. Bend left leg and take hold of its foot with left hand, and raise right arm as shown. Ease foot as close to seat as you can and hold for 8 counts. Slowly release, and repeat with other leg.

9. *Chest stretch*

Stand with feet a comfortable distance apart. Extend arms behind you and, clasping the hands, raise arms as high as possible. Hold for 8 counts.

10. Inner thigh and upper back stretch

Stand with feet wide apart with one foot turned out to the side slightly and the knee bent directly over that foot. Keep the other leg straight, with foot parallel. Extend both arms in front at shoulder level and clasp hands with palms facing outwards. Hold for 8 counts. Slowly straighten leg, then repeat to other side.

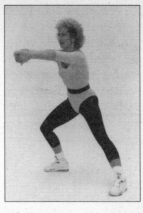

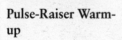

11. Tricep stretch

Stand with feet a comfortable distance apart and knees slightly bent. Ease one arm across chest holding it above the elbow with the other hand. Hold for 8 seconds. Slowly release, and repeat with other arm.

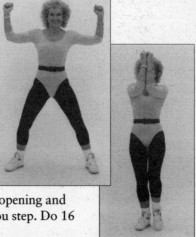

Pulse-Raiser Warm-up

Follow exercises 12–23 at low-impact level.

12. Side steps

Step from side to side, opening and closing bent arms as you step. Do 16 (8 each side).

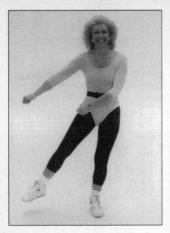

13. *Sideways jogging*
Jog from side to side, swinging arms as you go. Do 16.

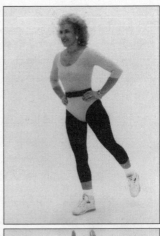

14. *Forward and backward jogging*
Stand with one leg in front of the other. Jog, transferring weight from one leg to the other, like a pendulum swinging. Do 16 with one leg in front, then change legs and repeat.

15. *Marching*
March on the spot and clap hands above head. Do 16 steps.

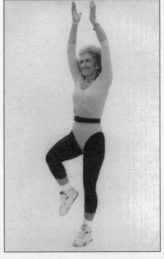

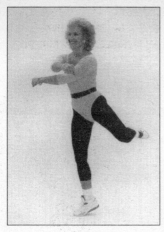

16. *Kick back*
Kick back with alternate feet, bending the knee as you kick and, at the same time, swinging arms out to sides and then crossing them in front. Do 16 (8 each foot).

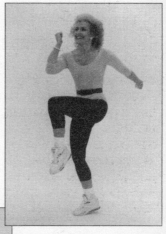

17. *Knee raises to opposite elbow*
Raise alternate knees towards opposite elbow. Do 16 (8 each knee).

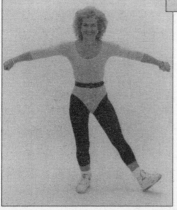

18. *Alternate heel digs to side*
Do 24 heel digs to alternate sides (12 each side), swinging arms out to sides and crossing them in front.

19. *Step and kick*
Step with one foot and kick across with the other foot, swinging arms to opposite side. Do 16 to alternate sides (8 each side).

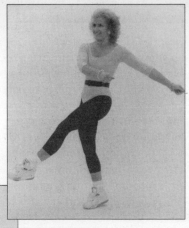

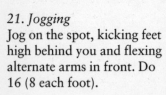

20. *Alternate heel digs, arm flexes*
Do 16 heel digs (8 each heel), alternating heels and at the same time flexing and straightening the arms.

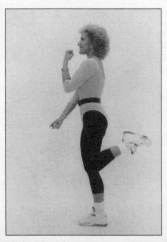

21. *Jogging*
Jog on the spot, kicking feet high behind you and flexing alternate arms in front. Do 16 (8 each foot).

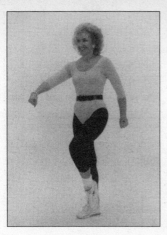

22. *Walking jog*
Walk on the spot, swinging arms as you step. Do 16 steps.

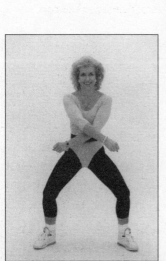

23. *Arm circles*
Standing with feet wide apart, swing both arms out and round in a full circle, crossing them in front and bending the knees as you swing. Do 8 inward circles and 8 outward circles.

Fat-Burner Workout

Repeat exercises 13–22 *twice* at high-impact level (or low-impact as necessary).

Cool Down

Repeat exercises 13–23 at low-impact level.

Repeat stretches 6–11.

DAY 8 DIET

Breakfast
1/2 oz (12.5 g) any cereal and 1 oz (25 g) All-Bran, plus milk from allowance and 1 teaspoon sugar.

Lunch
8 oz (200 g) jacket potato topped with 4 oz (100 g) baked beans.

Dinner
Coq au Vin (*see recipe*) served with vegetables of your choice, then Pineapple, Peach and Strawberry Dessert (*see recipe*).

With just six days to go you must be feeling a lot happier with the way you look and feel. Your holiday is just a few days away, so don't even think about cheating or letting up on the exercises. Every day is vital and one major lapse into overeating could seriously affect your progress. Be extra careful this week.

Have you made appointments with the hairdresser and the chiropodist? Having our hair trimmed just prior to going away means that we can manage it more easily. When you are at the hairdresser's ask for advice on the appropriate shampoo and conditioner to use while you are on holiday. There are now many different formulas to help protect the hair from the sunshine. Take a small bottle away with you – not an economy size.

Treating yourself to a chiropody treatment can make walking so much more comfortable. We want our feet to look good in our summer sandals, so have any hard skin or corns removed professionally and paint your toenails to make the feet look as pretty as possible. Break in any new shoes or sandals prior to departure. A blister caused by wearing new shoes can be extremely aggravating. I expect, if you are going to a warm climate you will not be wearing tights too often, but bare feet rub more easily and can become very sore. Just wearing new shoes around the house for an hour or so is sufficient to make them feel comfortable and problem-free.

Today's exercise programme is even more energetic. Try to do as much as you can at high-impact level within the peak aerobic section. You can always bring the pace down by going to low-impact in the middle of an exercise and then returning to high-impact when you feel able. Do ensure that the music you exercise to is really vibrant and fun. It is a great motivater and can increase the effectiveness of your exercises because, when the enjoyment level is raised appreciably, you can carry on for longer without feeling tired. In tests, athletes have been found to perform dramatically better when training to music.

The Mini Pizzas (*see recipe*) which are on your lunch menu today are a real treat. Those that are not used can be frozen to save time – and energy – later in the week. Fill up with lots of fresh crisp salad and look forward to your Savoury Oven-Baked Chicken Legs (*see recipe*) this evening.

It is important not to eat anything between meals, and once you get out of the habit, it becomes increasingly easier not to do so. This is the main reason why I have been able to maintain my weight in the last twelve months. I do not now feel hungry between meals because the question of whether I'm going to eat something or not never arises. Once this rule between the brain and the stomach had been established, I no longer suffered from any hunger pangs. It is a question of discipline and determination. I hope you will be able to establish this principle not only during the current 14-day period, but also during your holiday and when you return. Just as nibbling and overeating can become a habit, we are capable of educating our body to prevent over-indulgence.

After today there are only five more days on this diet to follow. Between now and the end of the week you can still lose a significant amount of weight, and some inches (cm), so please persevere and don't look back: look forward to day 15 and the final weighing and measuring session. Just go for it.

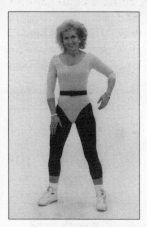

Mobilizing Warm-up

1. Shoulder rotations
Rotate alternate shoulders backwards 8 times, then forwards 8 times (4 each shoulder). Then repeat, rotating both shoulders together.

2. Alternate heel digs to side
Do 16 heel digs to alternate sides (8 each side), swinging arms out to sides and crossing them in front.

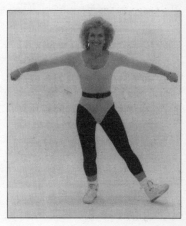

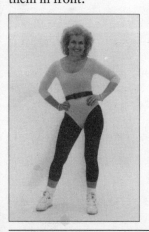

3. Alternate hip rotations
Rotate hips first in a clockwise direction, then in anti-clockwise direction. Repeat alternate hip rotations 8 times (4 each direction).

4. *Sideways curve*
Do 16 sideways curves to alternate sides (8 each side).

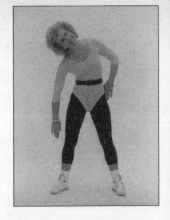

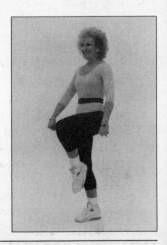

5. *Walking jog, arm circles*
Do a walking jog on the spot, circling alternate arms backwards as you step. Do 16 circles (8 each arm).

6. *Knee raises*
Raise alternate knees and at the same time draw hands forward and back, as if opening and closing a drawer. Do 24 raises (12 each knee).

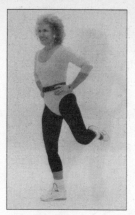

7. *Kick back*
Kick back with alternate feet, bending the knee as you kick. Do 24 (12 each foot).

Stretches

8. *Calf stretch*
Stand with feet parallel, one foot in front of the other. Keeping back leg straight and both heels on the floor, bend front knee as shown. Hold for 8 counts. Slowly release, and repeat with other leg in front.

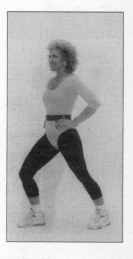

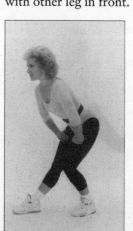

9. *Hamstring stretch*
Stand with feet parallel and hip-width apart, one foot in front of the other. Keep front leg straight and bend the knee of the other leg as shown ensuring that both heels remain on the floor. Hold for 8 counts. Raise the toes of the straight leg and hold for a further 8 counts. Slowly release, and repeat with other leg in front.

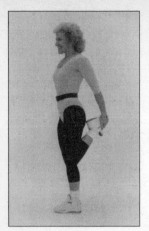

10. Front thigh stretch

Stand with feet together. Bend left leg and take hold of its foot with left hand as shown. Ease foot as close to seat as you can and hold for 8 counts. Slowly release, and repeat with other leg.

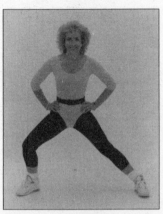

11. Inner thigh stretch

Stand with feet wide apart with one foot turned out to the side slightly and the knee bent directly over that foot. Keep the other leg straight, with foot parallel, and hold for 8 counts. Slowly straighten leg, then repeat to other side.

12. Tricep stretch

Stand with feet a comfortable distance apart and knees slightly bent. Ease one arm across chest holding it above the elbow with the other hand. Hold for 8 seconds. Slowly release, and repeat with other arm.

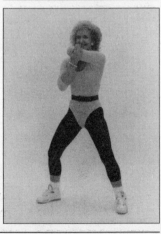

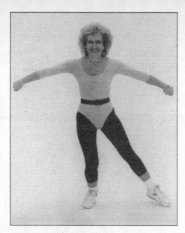

Pulse-Raiser Warm-up

Follow exercises 13–22 at low-impact level.

13. *Step and point*

Extend one leg out to the side, pointing the foot, and at the same time swing arms out to sides. Bring leg and arms in again, and repeat to the other side. Do 16 (8 each side).

14. *Kick back*

Kick back with alternate feet, bending the knee as you kick and, at the same time, swinging arms out to sides and then crossing them in front. Do 16 (8 each foot).

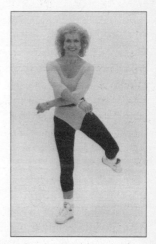

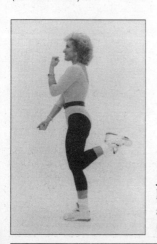

15. *Jogging*

Jog on the spot, kicking feet high behind you and flexing alternate arms in front. Do 16 (8 each foot).

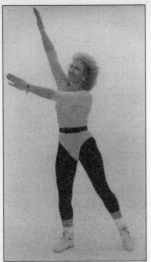

16. *Arm swinging*

Swing arms from side to side in a large sweeping movement, bending the knees and transferring weight from one foot to the other as you go. Do 16 (8 each side).

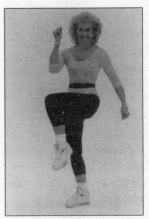

17. *Knee raises to opposite elbow*

Raise alternate knees towards opposite elbow. Do 16 (8 each knee).

18. *Kick back and touch*

Kick back with alternate feet to touch opposite hand behind you and swinging other arm as high as you can. Repeat 16 times (8 each foot).

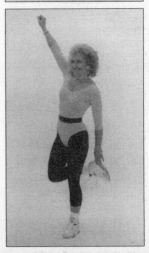

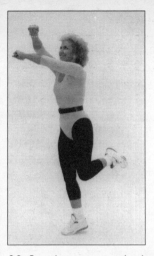

19. Kick back, arms high
Kick back with alternate feet, raising arms as you swing them out and across.

20. Jogging, arms swinging
Jog on the spot, swinging arms out to sides and then crossing them in front as you go. Do 16.

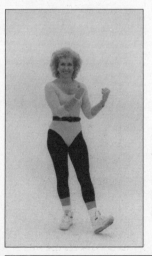

21. Alternate heel digs, arm flexes
Do 16 heel digs (8 each heel), alternating heels and at the same time flexing and straightening the arms.

22. Ski down

Stand with feet together, arms upstretched. Swing arms down to your sides, bending the knees as you go. Return to starting position and repeat, swinging arms up and down. Do 8.

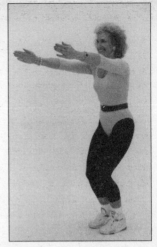

Fat-Burner Workout

Repeat exercises 13–21 *twice* at high-impact level (or low-impact as necessary).

Cool Down

Repeat exercises 13–22 at low-impact level.

Repeat stretches 8–12.

DAY 9 DIET

Breakfast
1 oz (25 g) toast spread with mustard and topped with 2oz (50 g) lean ham.

Lunch
1 Mini Pizza *(see recipe)* with salad.

Dinner
Savoury Oven-Baked Chicken Legs (*see recipe*) with vegetables of your choice, plus 5 oz (125 g) jacket potato or new potatoes, followed by Raspberry Surprise (*see recipe*).

Try on your skirt (or trousers) again this morning to check how much looser it feels. This should inspire you to keep on the straight and narrow throughout the day. Follow the exercises with extra vigour and, if you are inclined, increase the number of repetitions as you feel able.

Today's menus offer a variety of flavours and textures. Bran cereal mixed with sliced banana is a delightful combination, and if you've never tried cottage cheese with Marmite, you'll find that they make a delicious sandwich. The Marinated Lamb (*see recipe*) for this evening's dinner needs to be prepared well in advance. It constitutes a substantial meal and the prospect of fresh strawberries with yogurt to finish, brings the day to a satisfying conclusion.

As the days are ticking by, now is the time to check all the security arrangements for your home. Also start laying out your clothes ready to pack and do the main laundry session so that there is time for the clothes you wish to take away to be ironed and aired.

Add to your packing 'check list' any further items that you need to include in your luggage. Tick them off as you place them ready to be packed so that you feel totally in control of the whole planning and packing operation. It eases a great deal of stress as departure day draws nearer. Careful packing can prevent a great deal of creasing or damaged clothes. Having flown 85 times in the last four years, I speak from some personal experience! (See **Ten Tips for Perfect Packing** on page 189.) Overseas book promotional tours involve a great deal of flying, very little time in one place, and a change of clothes needs to be ready – often within minutes of arrival. Careful selection of colour co-ordinated outfits that are crease-resistant, combined with careful packing, can save many wasted minutes ironing. When you are on holiday, in particular, ironing is the last thing you want to be thinking about.

Enjoy the exercises and today's meals. Remember to choose one of the other menus if today's suggestions are inconvenient for you. Only four more days of dieting to go after today, so look forward and stick with it.

DAY 10 FAT-BURNER FITNESS PROGRAMME

Mobilizing Warm-up

1. Shoulder rotations
Rotate alternate shoulders backwards 8 times, then forwards 8 times (4 each shoulder). Then repeat, rotating both shoulders together.

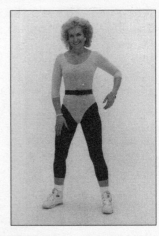

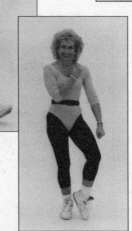

2. Heel digs, toe taps
Dig the heel and then tap the toe of one foot, while flexing alternate arms in front. Do 16 with one foot, then repeat with other foot.

3. *Walking jog, arm circles*

Do a walking jog on the spot, circling alternate arms backwards as you step. Do 16 circles (8 each arm).

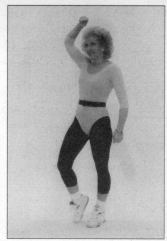

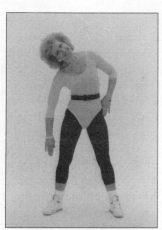

4. *Sideways curve*

Do 16 sideways curves to alternate sides (8 each side).

5. *Waist twist*

With knees slightly bent and elbows bent outwards at shoulder level, twist upper body to alternate sides. Do 16 to alternate sides (8 each side).

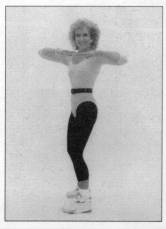

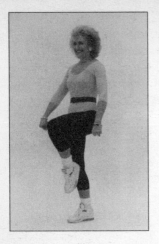

6. *Knee raises*

Raise alternate knees and at the same time draw hands forward and back, as if opening and closing a drawer. Do 16 raises (8 each knee).

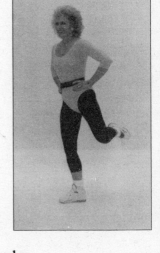

7. *Kick back*

Kick back with alternate feet, bending the knee as you kick. Do 24 (12 each foot).

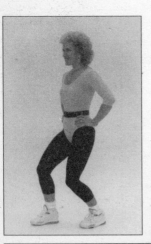

Stretches

8. *Calf stretch*

Stand as shown with feet parallel, one foot in front of the other. Keeping both heels on the floor, bend both knees and hold for 8 counts. Slowly release, and repeat with other leg in front.

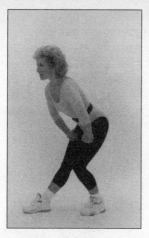

9. Hamstring stretch

Stand with feet parallel and hip-width apart, one foot in front of the other. Keep front leg straight and bend the knee of the other leg as shown ensuring that both heels remain on the floor. Hold for 8 counts. Raise the toes of the straight leg and hold for a further 8 counts. Slowly release, and repeat with other leg in front.

10. Front thigh stretch

Stand with feet together. Bend left leg and take hold of its foot with left hand as shown. Ease foot as close to seat as you can and hold for 8 counts. Slowly release, and repeat with other leg.

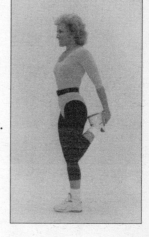

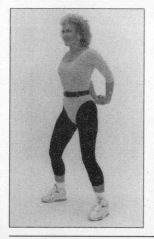

11. Chest stretch

Stand with feet a comfortable distance apart. Extend arms behind you and, clasping the hands, raise arms as high as possible. Hold for 8 counts.

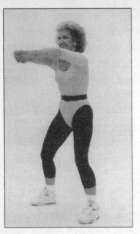

12. *Upper back stretch*
Stand with feet a comfortable distance apart, knees slightly bent. Extend both arms in front of you and clasp hands together. Hold for 8 counts.

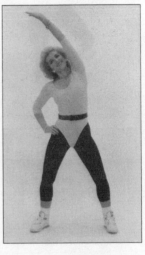

13. *Waist stretch*
Stand with feet a comfortable distance apart. Reach one arm over to side with palm of hand facing ceiling. Hold for 8 counts and repeat to other side.

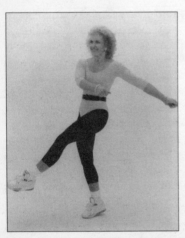

Pulse-Raiser Warm-up

Follow exercises 14–18 and 20–22 at low-impact level.

14. *Step and kick*
Step with one foot and kick across with the other foot, swinging arms to opposite side. Do 16 to alternate sides (8 each side).

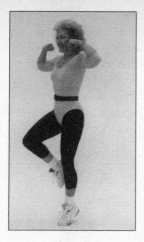

15. *Jogging, arm bends*
Jog on the spot, alternately bending and straightening arms out to sides at shoulder level. Do 16 steps.

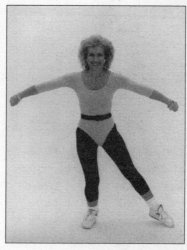

16. *Step and point*
Extend one leg out to the side, pointing the foot, and at the same time swing arms out to sides. Bring leg and arms in again, and repeat to other side. Do 16 (8 each side).

17. *Jogging, arms swinging*
Jog on the spot, swinging arms out to sides and then crossing them in front as you go. Do 16.

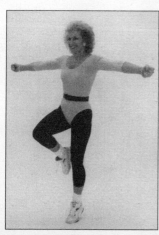

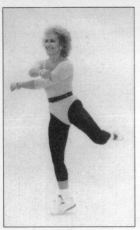

18. Kick back

Kick back with alternate feet, bending the knee as you kick and, at the same time, swinging arms out to sides and then crossing them in front. Do 16 (8 each foot).

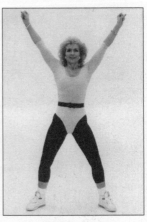

19. Jumping jacks

Jump, landing with feet apart, then jump again, landing with feet together. Raise and lower arms at your sides as you jump. Do 8.

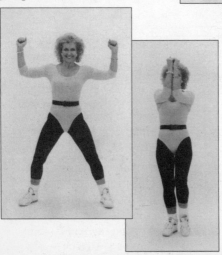

20. Side steps

Step from side to side, opening and closing bent arms as you step. Do 24 (12 each side).

21. *Jogging, arms flexing*
Jog on the spot, flexing alternate arms. Do 16.

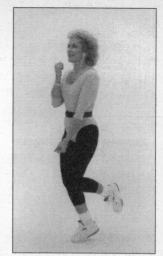

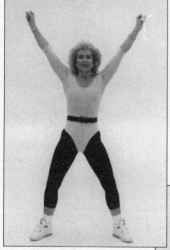

22. *Arm circles*
Standing with feet wide apart, swing both arms out and around in a full circle, crossing them in front and bending the knees as you swing. Do 8 inward circles and 8 outward circles.

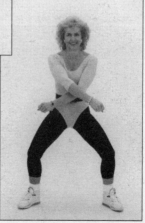

Fat-Burner Workout

Repeat exercises 14–21 *three times* at high-impact level (or low-impact as necessary).

Cool Down

Repeat exercises 14–18 and 20–22 at low-impact level.

Repeat stretches 8–13.

DAY 10 DIET

Breakfast
1¹/ oz (37.5 g) branflakes or All-Bran, plus a medium-sized, sliced banana, served with milk from allowance and 1 teaspoon brown sugar.

Lunch
2 slices (2 oz/50 g) bread spread with Marmite and filled with 4 oz (100 g) cottage cheese.

Dinner
Marinated Lamb (*see recipe*) with vegetables of your choice, plus 6 oz (150 g) fresh strawberries topped with 2 oz (50 g) diet strawberry yogurt.

If you have time, try to combine your fat-burner workout with some additional physical activity today. Either go to an exercise class, work out to a fitness video or play a game of your favourite sport. We want to try and be as energetic as possible as we reach the end of our 14-day Shape-Up for Summer programme.

Today's meals are very straightforward. If you want to make any of the menus more exciting, by all means pick one of the other recipes included in this book.

Today would be an ideal time to apply any overnight tanning cream that you plan to use. There is nothing worse than arriving at a sunny seaside resort with totally white legs and body. Never before have we had such a choice of good-quality, overnight tanning lotions. These will wear off after a few days, but they will take the edge off the whiteness for the first three days until the melanin in your skin reaches the surface and starts converting to a beautiful natural tan. Take the trouble to read my notes on tanning in the **Body Care** chapter. In the meantime, apply your overnight tan tonight, but ensure that you give it time to dry thoroughly before getting into bed – otherwise it may mark the sheets. Take extra care to wash your hands thoroughly after application as failing to do so will leave you with very brown hands and be a real give-away that your tan isn't natural!

Purchase any last-minute wardrobe or cosmetic items that are still outstanding. Also, check the first-aid kit (see page 190 for further advice) and buy any medications that you feel are appropriate to your holiday location.

Leave room in your suitcase for a beach ball and some other activity aids. Being as active as possible while away is the key to maintaining the magnificent weight loss you will have achieved over these two weeks. A blow-up beach ball takes up little space in a suitcase, yet can be a useful item to take on the beach not only to play games with the family, but also to use as a prop for the **Five-Minute Beach Workout** which I have included on page 207. These exercises are discreet and can be practised easily while you are sunning yourself.

Enjoy today's exercises and keep looking at yourself in the mirror to see how you're progressing. Have a great day.

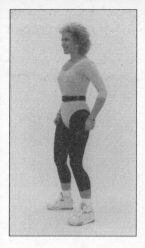

Mobilizing Warm-up

1. Shoulder rotations
Rotate both shoulders backwards 8 times, then forwards 8 times.

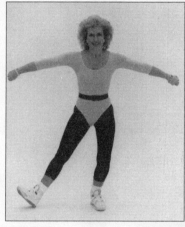

2. Alternate heel digs to side
Do 16 heel digs to alternate sides (8 each side), swinging arms out to sides and crossing them in front.

3. Alternate hip rotations
Rotate hips first in a clockwise direction, then in an anti-clockwise direction. Repeat alternate hip rotations 8 times (4 each direction).

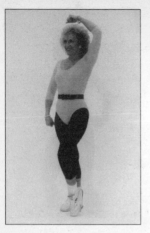

4. *Walking jog, arm circles*
Do a walking jog on the spot, circling alternate arms backwards as you step. Do 16 circles (8 each arm).

5. *Waist twist*
With knees slightly bent and elbows bent outwards at shoulder level, twist upper body to alternate sides. Do 16 to alternate sides (8 each side).

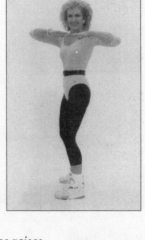

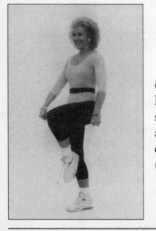

6. *Knee raises*
Raise alternate knees and at the same time draw hands forward and back, as if opening and closing a drawer. Do 16 raises (8 each knee).

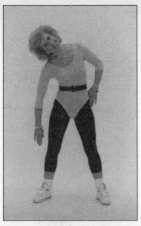

7. *Sideways curve*

Do 16 sideways curves to alternate sides (8 each side).

Stretches

8. *Hamstring stretch*

Stand with feet parallel and hip-width apart, one foot in front of the other. Keep front leg straight and bend the knee of the other leg as shown ensuring that both heels remain on the floor. Hold for 8 counts. Raise the toes of the straight leg and hold for a further 8 counts. Slowly release, and repeat with other leg in front.

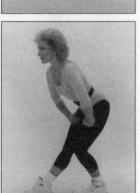

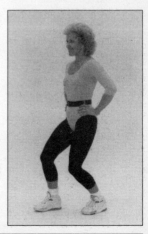

9. *Calf stretch*

Stand as shown with feet parallel, one foot in front of the other. Keeping both heels on the floor, bend both knees and hold for 8 counts. Slowly release, and repeat with other leg in front.

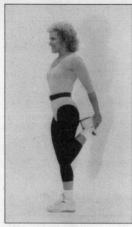

10. *Front thigh stretch*
Stand with feet together. Bend left leg and take hold of its foot with left hand as shown. Ease foot as close to seat as you can and hold for 8 counts. Slowly release, and repeat with other leg.

11. *Inner thigh and upper back stretch*
Stand with feet wide apart with one foot turned out to the side slightly and the knee bent directly over that foot. Keep the other leg straight, with foot parallel. Extend both arms in front at shoulder level and clasp hands with palms facing outwards. Hold for 8 counts. Slowly straighten leg, then repeat to other side.

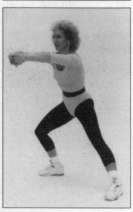

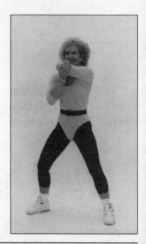

12. *Tricep stretch*
Stand with feet a comfortable distance apart and knees slightly bent. Ease one arm across chest holding its elbow with the other hand. Hold for 8 seconds. Slowly release, and repeat with other arm.

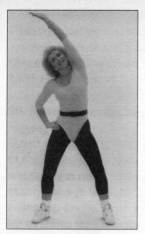

13. *Waist stretch*
Stand with feet a comfortable distance apart. Reach one arm over to side with palm of hand facing ceiling. Hold for 8 counts. Slowly release, and repeat to other side.

Pulse-Raiser Warm-up

Follow exercises 14–24 at low-impact level.

14. *Step and kick*
Step with one foot and kick across with the other foot, swinging arms to opposite side. Do 16 to alternate sides (8 each side).

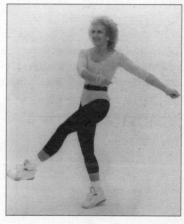

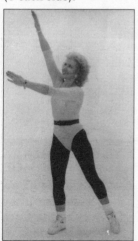

15. *Arm swinging*
Swing arms from side to side in a large sweeping movement, bending the knees and transferring weight from one foot to the other as you go. Do 16 (8 each side).

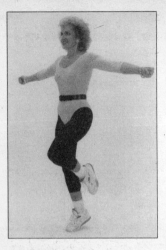

16. *Jogging, arm bends*
Jog on the spot, alternately bending and straightening arms out to sides at shoulder level. Do 16 steps.

17. *Jogging*
Jog on the spot, kicking feet high behind you and flexing alternate arms in front. Do 16 (8 each foot).

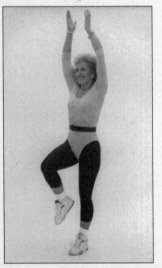

18. *Marching*
March on the spot and clap hands above head. Do 16 steps.

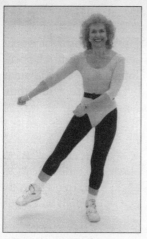

19. *Sideways jogging*
Jog from side to side, swinging arms as you go. Do 16.

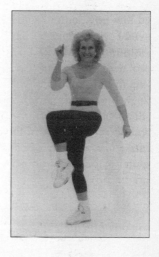

20. *Knee raises to opposite elbow*
Raise alternate knees towards opposite elbow. Do 16 (8 each knee).

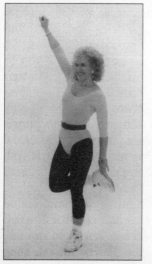

21. *Kick back and touch*
Kick back with alternate feet to touch opposite hand behind you and swinging other arm as high as you can. Repeat 16 times (8 each foot).

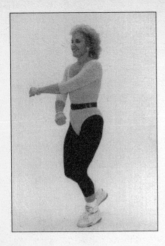

22. *Jogging, arms swinging*
Jog on the spot, swinging arms out to sides and then crossing them in front as you go. Do 24.

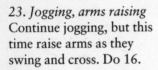

23. *Jogging, arms raising*
Continue jogging, but this time raise arms as they swing and cross. Do 16.

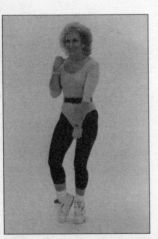

24. *Walking, arms flexing*
Walk on the spot, flexing alternate arms in front. Do 16 steps.

Fat-Burner Workout

Repeat exercises 14–24 three times at high-impact level (or low-impact as necessary).

Cool Down

Repeat exercises 14–24 at low-impact level

Repeat stretches 7–13.

DAY 11 DIET

Breakfast
2 oz (50 g) bread roll spread with 2 teaspoons marmalade or honey.

Lunch
3 oz (75 g) smoked mackerel with salad of grated carrot, beetroot and home-made Coleslaw (*see recipe*), plus 1 teaspoon horseradish.

Dinner
6 oz (150 g) chicken, cooked without fat and all skin removed, or 8 oz (200 g) white fish, steamed or microwaved, served with unlimited vegetables of your choice

or

Lemon Glazed Vegetables (*see recipe*), followed by a meringue basket filled with a petit fromage frais and topped with fresh raspberries or strawberries.

Well, you're nearly there. Only three more days of the diet to go. Be inspired to stick with the programme for the next three days – keep thinking about how great you're going to look on the beach this holiday. Buy lots of diet drinks to keep you satisfied in between meals, but if you feel really peckish at any time, then a raw carrot is probably the most harmless item of food to alleviate any hunger pangs.

Today's meals include a high-fibre breakfast, followed by rye crispbreads for lunch, topped with a choice of either cottage cheese or Smoked Mackerel Pâté (*see recipe*). The latter needs to be prepared in advance and makes a delicious lunch, but it can also be served as an hors d'oeuvre on a dinner-party menu. The Chicken and Potato Pie (*see recipe*) for this evening's meal is easy to prepare, while the Cheese and Apricot Pears (*see recipe*) makes a rather special dessert which should help you feel content with the diet as opposed to feeling deprived.

Work out with extra energy today. You should be feeling significantly fitter than you did on Day 1 and your body must be in dramatically better shape as a result. Also, play some new music and make sure that it has a strong beat and an inspirational sound.

Well done for getting this far. The winning post is almost in sight so don't even consider wavering from the diet or exercise programme.

DAY 12 FAT-BURNER FITNESS PROGRAMME

Mobilizing Warm-up

1. Shoulder rotations
Rotate both shoulders
backwards 8 times, then
forwards 8 times.

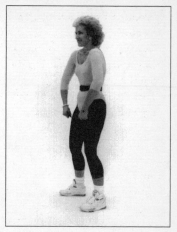

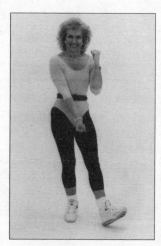

2. Heel digs, toe taps
Dig the heel and then tap the
toe of one foot, while flexing
alternate arms in front. Do
16 with one foot, then repeat
with other foot.

3. Alternate hip rotations
Rotate hips first in a
clockwise direction, then
in an anti-clockwise
direction. Repeat alternate
hip rotations 8 times (4
each direction).

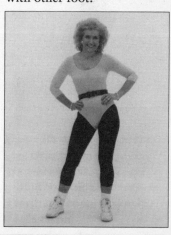

4. Sideways curve

Do 16 sideways curves to alternate sides (8 each side).

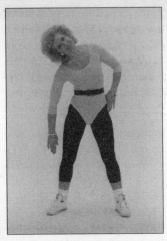

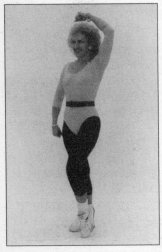

5. Walking jog, arm circles

Do a walking jog on the spot, circling alternate arms backwards as you step. Do 16 circles (8 each arm).

6. Kick back

Kick back with alternate feet, bending the knee as you kick. Do 24 (12 each foot).

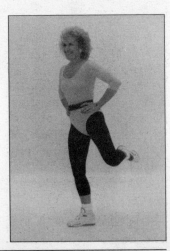

7. *Waist twist*

With knees slightly bent and elbows bent outwards at shoulder level, twist upper body to alternate sides. Do 16 to alternate sides (8 each side).

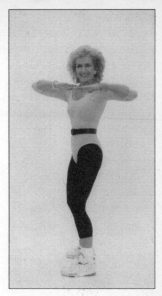

Stretches

8. *Hamstring stretch*

Stand with feet parallel and hip-width apart, one foot in front of the other. Keep front leg straight and bend the knee of the other leg as shown, ensuring that both heels remain on the floor. Hold for 8 counts. Raise the toes of the straight leg and hold for a further 8 counts. Slowly release, and repeat with other leg in front.

9. *Calf stretch*

Stand as shown with feet parallel, one foot in front of the other. Keeping both heels on the floor, bend both knees and hold for 8 counts. Slowly release, and repeat with other leg in front.

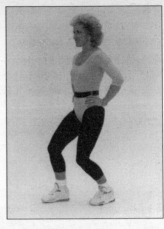

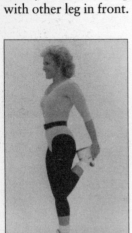

10. *Front thigh stretch*

Stand with feet together. Bend left leg and take hold of its foot with left hand as shown. Ease foot as close to seat as you can and hold for 8 counts. Slowly release, and repeat with other leg.

11. *Chest stretch*

Stand with feet a comfortable distance apart. Extend arms behind you and, clasping the hands, raise arms as high as possible. Hold for 8 counts.

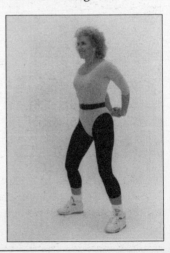

12. *Waist stretch*
Stand with feet a comfortable distance apart. Reach one arm over to side with palm of hand facing ceiling. Hold for 8 counts. Slowly release and repeat to other side.

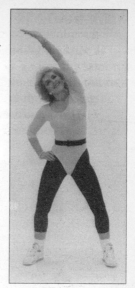

Pulse-Raiser Warm-up

Follow exercises 13–21 at low-impact level

13. *Step and point*
Extend one leg out to the side, pointing the foot, and at the same time swing arms out to sides. Bring leg and arms in again, and repeat to the other side. Do 16 (8 each side).

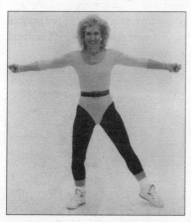

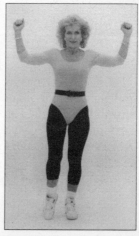

14. *Walking jog, arms in and out*
Walk on the spot, swinging bent arms in and out at shoulder level. Do 16.

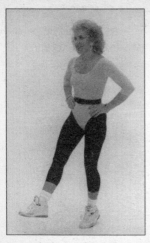

15. Forward and backward jogging

Stand with one leg in front of the other. Jog, transferring weight from one leg to the other, like a pendulum swinging. Do 16 with one leg in front, then change legs and repeat.

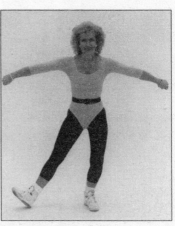

16. Alternate heel digs to side

Do 16 heel digs to alternate sides (8 each side), swinging arms out to sides and crossing them in front.

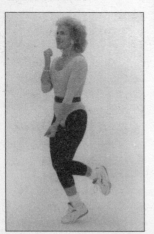

17. Jogging, arms flexing

Jog on the spot, flexing alternate arms. Do 16.

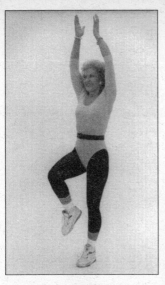

18. Marching
March on the spot and clap hands above head. Do 24 steps.

19. Jogging, arm bends
Jog on the spot, alternately bending and straightening arms out to sides at shoulder level. Do 16 steps.

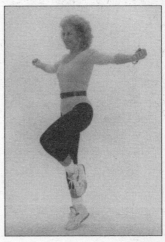

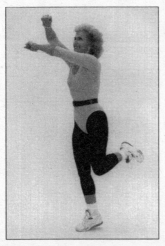

20. Kick back, arms high
Kick back with alternate feet, bending the knee as you kick and, at the same time, swinging arms out to sides and then crossing them in front of you at shoulder level. Do 16 (8 each foot).

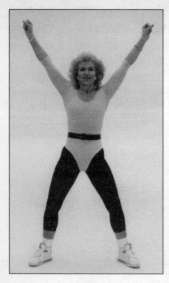

21. *Arm circles*
Standing with feet wide apart, swing both arms out and around in a full circle, crossing them in front and bending the knees as you swing. Do 8 inward circles and 8 outward circles.

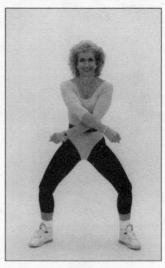

Fat-Burner Workout

Repeat exercises 13–20 at high-impact level (or low-impact as necessary).

Cool Down

Repeat exercises 13–16, 19 and 21 *twice* at low-impact level.

Repeat stretches 7–12.

DAY 12 DIET

Breakfast
1 oz (25 g) All-Bran and 1/2 oz (12.5 g) Fruit and
Fibre, plus milk from allowance and 1 teaspoon
sugar.

Lunch
4 Ryvitas spread with Marmite or Reduced-Oil
Salad Dressing (*see recipe*) and topped with either
cottage cheese or Smoked Mackerel Pâté (*see
recipe*).

Dinner
Chicken and Potato Pie (*see recipe*), then Cheese
and Apricot Pears (*see recipe*).

Today you can start packing but before you pack your swimsuit (or bikini), pop it on and see how different you look in the mirror. Put it on first thing in the morning before you've eaten anything and try to recall how you looked on that very first day. If you are in any doubt as to the progress that you've made, try on your skirt (or trousers) and realize how many inches (cm) you have lost.

Today's breakfast is a bit of a treat as the flavours of baked beans and bacon combine to make a delicious meal. The Chinese Salad (*see recipe*) is mega-filling and will satisfy any palate. It is also extremely rich in vitamins and other nutrients. The evening meal is ideal for vegetarians, but tempting enough for anyone to try. Fill up with lots of low-calorie vegetables and finish with fresh fruit salad topped with fromage frais.

With just one more workout after today, put an extra spring in your step and do as many repetitions of the fat-burner workout as you can manage. Also, today is the best day to do a blitz on the housework so that all will be clean and tidy when you return.

Check through all the items that you plan to take on holiday with you and carefully consider which clothes you might not wear and that could be left behind. We almost always take more away with us than we need and now is the time to fine-tune your packing list so that nothing unnecessary is taken. Having established that all that you plan to take is essential and will definitely be worn, pack any item which won't crease or that you do not need between now and departure date. Obviously, cosmetics and toiletries are last-minute items, but a great deal of progress can be made if you pack shoes, handbags, jewellery, T-shirts, shorts, swimwear and general accessories at this stage.

Remember to collect your travellers' cheques and any other outstanding documentation today, as tomorrow is likely to be very busy as you finalize such arrangements as who will be visiting the house to look after the plants, depositing pets at their carers and taking care of home security in general.

Go through your 'check list' again and make sure there is nothing else that you need to buy as tomorrow is your last day. Stick with the diet and do the exercises – the finishing post is now clearly in sight.

DAY 13 FAT-BURNER FITNESS PROGRAMME

Mobilizing Warm-up

1. Shoulder rotations
Rotate alternate shoulders backwards 8 times, then forwards 8 times (4 each shoulder). Then repeat, rotating both shoulders together.

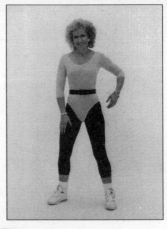

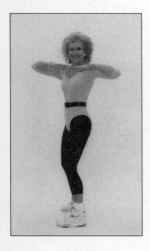

2. Waist twist
With knees slightly bent and elbows bent outwards at shoulder level, twist upper body to alternate sides. Do 16 to alternate sides (8 each side).

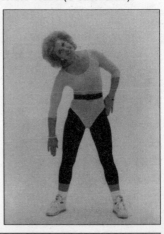

3. Sideways curve
Do 16 sideways curves to alternate sides
(8 each side).

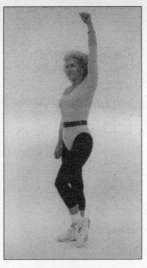

4. *Walking jog, arm circles*

Walk on the spot, swinging one arm backwards in a large circle 4 times. Repeat with other arm. Repeat, circling alternate arms forwards 8 times (4 each arm).

5. *Alternate heel digs to side*

Do 16 heel digs to alternate sides (8 each side), swinging arms out to sides and crossing them in front.

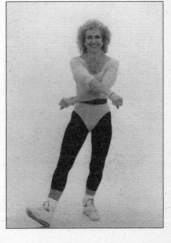

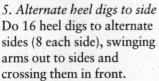

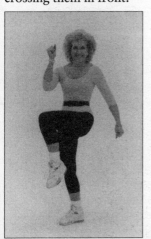

6. *Knee raises to opposite elbow*

Raise alternate knees towards opposite elbow. Do 16 (8 each knee).

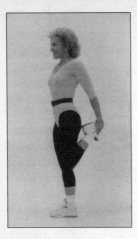

Stretches

7. *Front thigh stretch*
Stand with feet together. Bend left leg and take hold of its foot with left hand as shown. Ease foot as close to seat as you can and hold for 8 counts. Slowly release, and repeat with other leg.

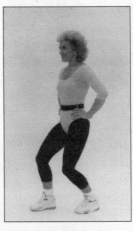

8. *Calf stretch*
Stand as shown with feet parallel, one foot in front of the other. Keeping both heels on the floor, bend both knees and hold for 8 counts. Slowly release, and repeat with other leg in front.

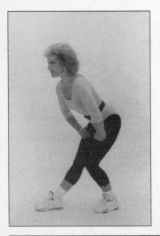

9. *Hamstring stretch*
Stand with feet parallel and hip-width apart, one foot in front of the other. Keep front leg straight and bend the knee of the other leg as shown ensuring that both heels remain on the floor. Hold for 8 counts. Raise the toes of the straight leg and hold for a further 8 counts. Slowly release, and repeat with other leg in front.

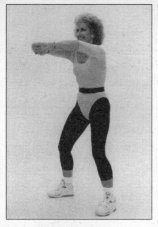

10. Upper back stretch
Stand with feet a comfortable distance apart, knees slightly bent. Extend both arms in front of you and clasp hands together. Hold for 8 counts.

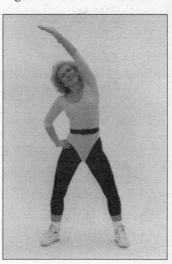

11. Waist stretch
Stand with feet a comfortable distance apart. Reach one arm over to side with palm of hand facing ceiling. Hold for 8 counts. Slowly release, and repeat to other side.

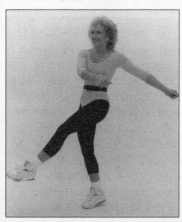

Pulse-Raiser Warm-up

Follow exercises 12–18, 20 and 22 at low-impact level.

12. Step and kick
Step with one foot and kick across with the other foot, swinging arms to opposite side. Do 16 to alternate sides (8 each side).

13. Jogging, arm bends

Jog on the spot, alternately bending and straightening arms out to sides at shoulder level. Do 16 steps.

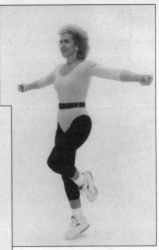

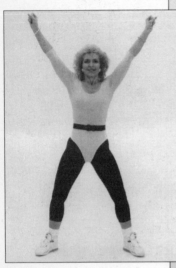

14. Jumping jacks

Jump, landing with feet apart, then jump again, landing with feet together. Raise and lower arms at your sides as you jump. Do 12.

15. Knee raises, arms out and in

Raise alternate knees, bringing bent arms out and in at shoulder level. Do 16

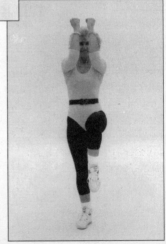

16. *Kick back*

Kick back with alternate feet, bending the knee as you kick and, at the same time, swinging arms out to sides and then crossing them in front. Do 16 (8 each foot).

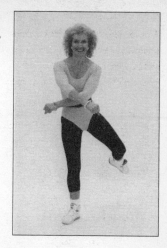

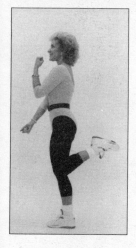

17. *Jogging*

Jog on the spot, kicking feet high behind you and flexing alternate arms in front. Do 16 (8 each foot).

18. *Arm swinging*

Swing arms from side to side in a large sweeping movement, bending the knees and transferring weight from one foot to the other as you go. Do 16 (8 each side).

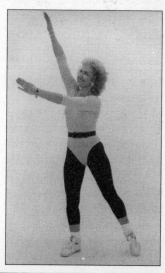

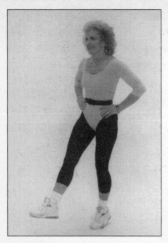

19. Forward and backward jogging
Stand with one leg in front of the other. Jog, transferring weight from one leg to the other, like a pendulum swinging. Do 16 with one leg in front, then change legs and repeat.

20. Alternate heel digs, arm flexes
Do 16 heel digs (8 each heel), alternating heels and at the same time flexing and straightening the arms.

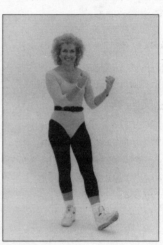

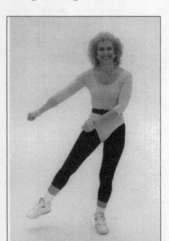

21. Sideways jogging
Jog from side to side, swinging arms as you go. Do 16.

22. Heel digs, toe taps

Dig the heel and then tap the toe of one foot, while flexing alternate arms in front. Do 16 with one foot, then repeat with other foot.

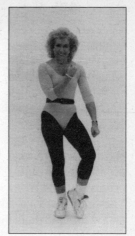

Fat-Burner Workout

Repeat exercises 12–22 three times at high-impact level (or low impact as necessary).

Cool Down

Repeat exercises 12–13, 15–18, 20 and 22 at low-impact level.

Repeat stretches 7–11.

DAY 13 DIET

Breakfast
1 oz (25 g) toast topped with 5 oz (125 g) baked beans, plus 1 oz (25 g) well grilled lean bacon.

Lunch
Chinese Salad (*see recipe*), plus 1 piece any fresh fruit.

Dinner
Cauliflower and Courgette Bake (*see recipe*) served with 4 oz (100 g) jacket potato, unlimited carrots and mange-tout, followed by 4 oz (100 g) fresh fruit salad topped with 3 oz (75 g) fromage frais.

Congratulations on reaching Day 14 of this day-by-day Shape-Up for Summer programme. It takes an enormous amount of willpower to stick with a programme of diet and exercise for 14 days and if you have adhered to it very carefully I am sure you will now be feeling that it was all worthwhile.

Today will be devoted to final arrangements and packing. If you are taking your dog to kennels or your cat to a cattery, ensure that you give the owner the telephone number and address of your regular vet in case of an emergency. This is particularly important if your dog or cat suffers from any recurring ailment or is old. Also, leave with them the details of your holiday address and, if possible, the address of a relative or friend who knows the animal and who could be called in to help if things become difficult.

Remember to cancel your milk and to check that a neighbour will keep an eye on the house so that any free newspapers left sticking out of the letter-box can be pushed through or any unexpected parcels collected from your doorstep. Ensure that the plants are properly watered and that your shed and garage are locked.

Today's meals have been specifically designed in the hope that you will weigh as little as possible for tomorrow morning's final weighing and measuring session. If you are planning to leave early, bring forward the session to today. Remember to pack your tape measure so that you can keep an eye on your measurements and check that not too much damage is being done while you are away.

Try to find time to do your final fat-burner workout which is particularly energetic today.

Last thing this evening do your final packing, but do not close the suitcase as this will unnecessarily squash the clothes. Leave all your toiletries and cosmetics out tonight so that after you've used them they can be simply slipped into a sponge or cosmetic bag as appropriate. Remember to keep a limited supply of essential items, e.g. toothbrush, deodorant, basic make-up, in your hand luggage in case of unavoidable delays caused by the airline. Also, pack a spare set of underwear for all of you, just in case your baggage gets delayed or misrouted. Gather together a few items to entertain you and your family while you are waiting at the airport.

You are now virtually at the end of your 14-day campaign. Tomorrow you are going away and your holiday begins. The enjoyment value should be twice as great as a result of making this effort over the last 14 days. Feeling happy about our body when we go away makes an enormous difference to how we feel about ourselves and how we react to the rest of the family. I hope your family recognizes all the hard work that you have put in and will support you throughout the holiday. Have a wonderful time and try to follow the guidelines included in chapters 6, 7 and 8 which will help you minimize the damage to your waistline while you're on holiday. *Bon voyage!*

DAY 14 FAT-BURNER FITNESS PROGRAMME

Mobilizing Warm-up

1. Shoulder rotations
Rotate both shoulders backwards
8 times, then forwards 8 times.

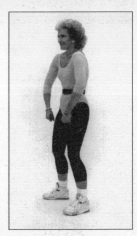

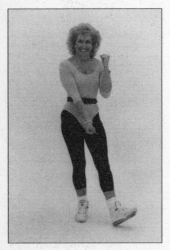

2. Heel digs, toe taps
Dig the heel and then tap
the toe of one foot, while
flexing alternate arms in
front. Do 16 with one foot,
then repeat with other foot.

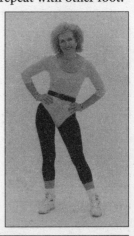

3. Alternate hip rotations
Rotate hips first in a clockwise
direction, then in an anti-
clockwise direction. Repeat
alternate hip rotations 8 times (4
each direction).

4. Sideways curve
Do 16 sideways curves to alternate sides (8 each side).

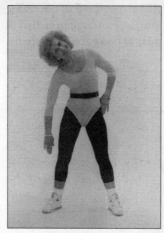

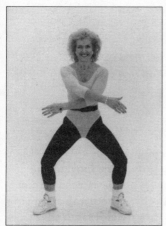

5. Arm circles
Standing with feet wide apart, swing both arms out and around in a full circle, crossing them in front and bending the knees as you swing. Do 8 inward circles and 8 outward circles.

6. Knee raises to opposite elbow
Raise alternate knees towards opposite elbow. Do 16 (8 each knee).

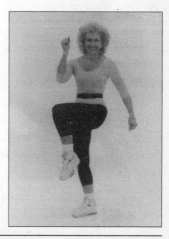

Stretches

7. *Calf stretch*

Stand as shown with feet parallel, one foot in front of the other. Keeping both heels on the floor, bend both knees and hold for 8 counts. Slowly release, and repeat with other leg in front.

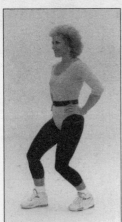

8. *Hamstring stretch*

Stand with feet parallel and hip-width apart, one foot in front of the other. Keep front leg straight and bend the knee of the other leg as shown ensuring that both heels remain on the floor. Hold for 8 counts. Raise the toes of the straight leg and hold for a further 8 counts. Slowly release, and repeat with other leg in front.

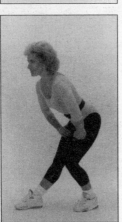

9. *Front thigh stretch*

Stand with feet together. Bend left leg and take hold of its foot with left hand as shown. Ease foot as close to seat as you can and hold for 8 counts. Slowly release, and repeat with other leg.

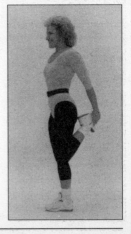

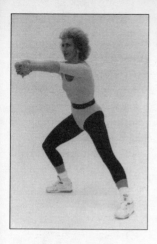

10. Inner thigh and upper back stretch

Stand with feet wide apart with one foot turned out to the side slightly and the knee bent directly over that foot. Keep the other leg straight, with foot parallel. Extend both arms in front at shoulder level and clasp hands with palms facing outwards. Hold for 8 counts. Slowly straighten leg, then repeat to other side.

11. Chest stretch

Stand with feet a comfortable distance apart. Extend arms behind you and, clasping the hands, raise arms as high as possible. Hold for 8 counts.

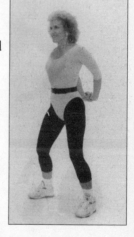

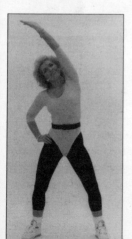

12. Waist stretch

Stand with feet a comfortable distance apart. Reach one arm over to side with palm of hand facing ceiling. Hold for 8 counts. Slowly release, and repeat to other side.

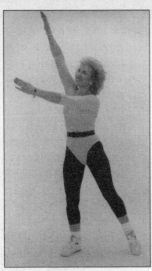

Pulse-Raiser Warm-up

Follow exercises 13–23 at low-impact level.

13. *Arm swinging*
Swing arms from side to side, bending the knees and transferring weight from one foot to the other as you go. Do 16 (8 each side).

14. *Jogging, arm bends*
Jog on the spot, alternately bending and straightening arms to the front of you at shoulder level. Do 16.

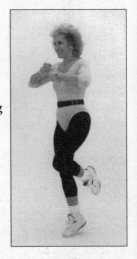

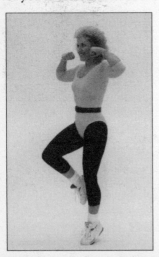

15. *Jogging, arm bends*
Continue jogging, but this time bending and straightening arms to the front *above* shoulder level. Do 16.

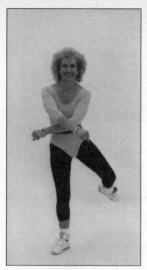

16. *Kick back*
Kick back with alternate feet, bending the knee as you kick, and at the same time swinging arms out to sides and then crossing them in front. Do 16 (8 each foot).

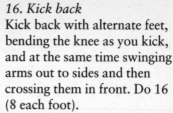

17. *Marching*
March on the spot and clap hands above head. Do 24 steps.

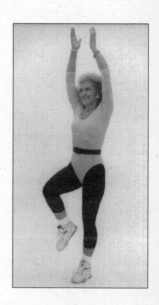

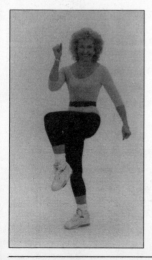

18. *Knee raises to opposite elbow*
Raise alternate knees towards opposite elbow. Do 16 (8 each knee).

19. Forward and backward jogging
Stand with one leg in front of the other. Jog, transferring weight from one leg to the other, like a pendulum swinging. Do 16 with one leg in front, then change legs and repeat.

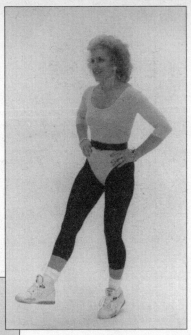

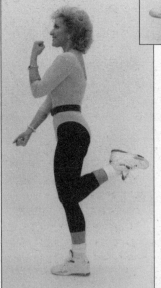

20. Jogging
Jog on the spot, kicking feet high behind you and flexing alternate arms in front. Do 16 (8 each foot).

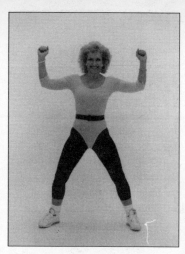

21. Side steps
Step from side to side, opening and closing bent arms as you step. Do 24 (12 each side).

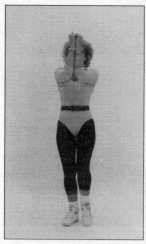

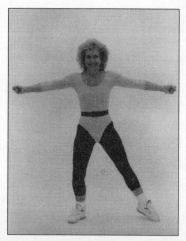

22. Step and point
Extend one leg out to the side, pointing the foot, and at the same time swing arms out to sides. Bring leg and arms in again, and repeat to the other side. Do 16 (8 each side).

23. *Walking jog, arms in and out*
Walk on the spot, swinging arms in and out to the front of you, keeping them below shoulder level.

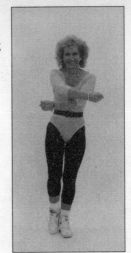

Fat-Burner Workout

Repeat exercises 13–23 *three times* at high-impact level (or low-impact as necessary).

Cool Down

Repeat exercises 13–23 at low-impact level.

Repeat stretches 7–12.

DAY 14 DIET

Breakfast
1 petit fromage frais, plus 2 pieces any fresh fruit.

Lunch
4 oz (100 g) chicken with large salad and 1 dessertspoon pickle.

Dinner
Poached Trout with Cucumber Sauce (*see recipe*) with green salad and 4 oz (100 g) new potatoes, plus Red Fruit Salad (*see recipe*).

2

14-Day Free Choice Diet

Daily Allowance:

5 fl oz (125 ml) unsweetened fruit juice
10 fl oz (250 ml) skimmed or semi-skimmed milk
1 alcoholic drink per day for women
2 alcoholic drinks per day for men

Select each day:

1 Breakfast menu
1 Lunch menu
1 Dinner (main course) menu
1 Dessert menu

BREAKFASTS

1. 1 oz (25 g) any cereal mixed with 5 oz (125 g) natural yogurt, plus 1 teaspoon sugar.

2. 12 oz (300 g) fresh fruit, or as much fruit as you can eat at one sitting.

3. 1 oz (25 g) porridge oats, cooked in water. Leave to stand overnight. Serve with 5 fl oz (125 ml) milk and 1 teaspoon honey or brown sugar.

4. 5 oz (125 g) natural yogurt, plus 1 teaspoon honey, topped with 2 teaspoons branflakes.

5. 1 banana chopped and 1 teaspoon strawberry preserve stirred into 5 oz (125 g) natural yogurt.

6. 1 oz (25 g) toast topped with 8 oz (200 g) baked beans.

7. 2 oz (50 g) toasted wholemeal bread spread with 3 teaspoons marmalade, honey or preserve.

8. 1½ oz (37.5 g) branflakes plus a medium-sized, sliced banana, served with milk from allowance and 1 teaspoon brown sugar.

9. 1 slice wholemeal toast spread with 2 teaspoons marmalade, plus 5 oz (125 g) diet yogurt – any flavour.

10. 1 oz (25 g) any cereal served with 5 fl oz (125 ml) semi-skimmed milk, plus 10 sultanas.

11. 1 oz (25 g) toast spread with 8 oz (200 g) tinned tomatoes – boil fast to reduce liquid and season well – topped with 1 oz (25 g) [cooked weight] lean bacon.

12. 8 oz (200 g) any tinned fruit in natural juice, plus 1 diet yogurt.

13. 1 petit fromage frais, 1 piece any fruit, 1 slice Slimcea or Nimble, plus 1 teaspoon jam, marmalade or honey.

14. 6 prunes, soaked in hot tea overnight, topped with 2 teaspoons natural yogurt.

LUNCHES

1. Select any four items from this list:

> 1 slimmers' cup-a-soup
> 1 diet yogurt
> 1 piece fresh fruit
> 1 low-fat fromage frais
> 2 rye crispbreads
> 2 oz (50 g) cottage cheese

2. 2 slices (2 oz/50 g total weight) wholemeal toast topped with 5 oz (125 g) baked beans, plus 2 grilled tomatoes.

3. 3 oz (75 g) smoked mackerel, tuna or salmon, served with large mixed salad and 2 oz (50 g) natural yogurt mixed with 1 teaspoon horseradish sauce.

Jacket potato lunches

4. 6 oz (150 g) jacket potato topped with one of the following, plus unlimited salad and soy sauce:

   2 oz (50 g) cottage cheese mixed with chopped peppers, pineapple, or chives;

   > *or*

   2 oz (50 g) baked beans;

   > *or*

   2 oz (50 g) sweetcorn mixed with 1 tablespoon Reduced-Oil Salad Dressing (*see recipe*);

   > *or*

   1 oz (25 g) cold chopped chicken mixed with natural yogurt and freshly ground black pepper;

   > *or*

   2 oz (50 g) prawns added to a mixture of 2 tablespoons natural yogurt, 1 tablespoon Reduced-Oil Salad Dressing (*see recipe*) and 1 tablespoon tomato ketchup.

Sandwich lunches

5. 3 slices (3 × 1 oz/25 g) bread, spread with Reduced-Oil Salad Dressing (*see recipe*) made into sandwiches with one of the following fillings:

   Carrot and Sultana Salad (*see recipe*) and 2 oz (50 g) cottage cheese;

or

sliced beetroot, onion and tomatoes, plus 1 teaspoon horseradish sauce;

or

2 oz (50 g) cottage cheese, plus lettuce, tomato and cucumber.

6. 3 slices (3 × 1 oz/25 g) bread, spread with natural yogurt and 1 teaspoon jam, made into sandwiches with a thinly sliced banana.

7. 2 slices (2 × 1 oz/25 g) bread, spread with mustard and/or pickle, made into sandwiches with one of the following:

2 oz (50 g) lean ham (all fat removed) and salad;

or

2 oz (50 g) chicken or turkey (no skin) and salad;

or

1½ oz (37.5 g) lean beef, plus sliced tomatoes.

8. 2 slices (2 × 1 oz/25 g) bread spread with Marmite and filled with 4 oz (100 g) cottage cheese. Add grated carrot if desired.

Salad lunches

9. Large salad comprising any of the following in unlimited quantities: lettuce, tomatoes, cucumber, sliced onion, chives, celery, grated carrot, beetroot, watercress, spinach, mushrooms – all prepared and served without oil – plus one of the following:

3 oz (75 g) chicken (no skin);

or

3 oz (75 g) turkey (no skin);

or

6 oz (150 g) prawns;

or

3 oz (75 g) lean ham (all fat removed);

or

2 oz (50 g) lean beef (all fat removed);

or

6 oz (150 g) cottage cheese;

or

3 oz (75 g) cottage cheese and 1 oz (25 g) lean ham or chicken;

or

3 oz (75 g) cold baked beans and 3 oz (75 g) cottage cheese.

Add mustard and/or 2 teaspoons sweet pickle if desired, plus 1 tablespoon Reduced-Oil Salad Dressing (*see recipe*) or unlimited fat-free sauce, e.g. soy sauce, Worcestershire sauce, Oil-Free Vinaigrette Dressing (*see recipe*) or natural yogurt.

Soup lunches

10. 1 tin (15 oz/375 g) any branded soup, except 'cream' varieties, plus 1 slice (1 oz/25 g) bread or toast.

11. 1/2 pint (250 ml) home-made soup (cooked without fat), plus 1 bread roll (2 oz/50 g).

DINNERS

1. 6 oz (150 g) chicken, cooked without fat and all skin removed, served with unlimited vegetables, restricting potatoes to 5 oz (125 g).

2. 8 oz (200 g) any white fish, steamed or microwaved, served with unlimited vegetables and low-fat parsley sauce (for cooking instructions, see introductory notes to **Day 5**) or tomato sauce.

3. 4 oz (100 g) grilled red meat (all fat removed), served with unlimited vegetables, plus gravy made without fat.

4. Beef and Mushroom Kebabs – 1 skewer per person (*see recipe* under **Barbecue Specials**.

5. Pork and Apricot Kebabs – 1 skewer per person (*see recipe* under **Barbecue Specials**), served with 4 oz (100 g) [cooked weight] boiled brown rice.

6. Surf 'n' Turf – 1 skewer per person (*see recipe* under **Barbecue Specials**), served with small jacket potato and salad.

7. Liver and Bacon Kebabs – 1 skewer per person (*see recipe* under **Barbecue Specials**), served with 4 oz (100 g) [cooked weight] boiled brown rice.

8. Chicken Curry (*see recipe*), served with 4 oz (100 g) [cooked weight] boiled brown rice.

9. Chicken and Mushroom Supreme (*see recipe*), served with unlimited vegetables and 4 oz (100 g) [cooked weight] boiled brown rice.

10. 6 oz (150 g) chicken breast, cooked in a packet casserole mix and served with unlimited vegetables.

11. Chicken Spaghetti – quick version – (*see recipe*).

12. 1 low-fat 'diet' prepacked meal, served with unlimited vegetables.

13. 6 oz (150 g) liver, braised with onions and served with unlimited vegetables.

14. 1 trout stuffed with prawns and served with unlimited vegetables.

DESSERTS

1. 2 pieces or 8 oz (200 g) any fresh fruit.

2. 5 oz (125 g) yogurt or fromage frais.

3. 6 oz (150 g) melon, chopped and mixed with melon-flavoured, low-fat yogurt.

4. 2 Ryvitas, plus 2 oz (50 g) cottage cheese and celery.

5. 4 oz (100 g) fresh fruit salad, plus 3 oz (75 g) diet yogurt.

6. 5 oz (125 g) strawberry-flavoured yogurt mixed with half a chopped banana.

7. 1 meringue basket filled with low-fat fromage frais and topped with 4 oz (100 g) fruit of your choice.

8. Mango and Strawberry Bombe (*see recipe*).

9. Raspberry Delight (*see recipe*).

10. Red Fruit Salad (*see recipe*).

11. 8 oz (200 g) strawberries or raspberries, plus 1 dessert-spoon diet yogurt.

12. 1 sliced fresh peach, plus 1 oz (25 g) non-Cornish ice cream.

13. 3 oz (75 g) frozen yogurt.

14. 1½ oz non-Cornish ice cream.

3

Body Care

A light tan and sun-kissed hair is a look many of us may hope to achieve as summer approaches. However, the summer months can be quite harsh on the body, causing the skin and hair to become dry and lacking in natural lustre.

The main source of damage is the sun. Excessive exposure to the sun's rays can result in serious damage to the skin, causing premature ageing and increasing the risk of contracting skin cancer. The good news is that there is now a plentiful supply of excellent self-tanning products on the market that can help us acquire the look we desire without putting our health – or our looks – at risk. However, for those of us who still wish to acquire a natural tan, with adequate preparation and sensible precautions a great deal of harm can be prevented.

Sunshine is a source of Vitamin D – which is important for those on a low-fat diet. Vitamin D is found in margarine and various other foods which are omitted from or greatly reduced on a low-fat diet. However, Vitamin D is a fat-soluble vitamin and can be stored in the body for several months, so we are unlikely to become deficient if we stock up during the summer months.

Suntanning

Preparation for your tan should start as early as possible. At least two weeks prior to your holiday, apply a moisturizing body lotion after every bath or shower. This helps the skin to stay soft and moist and will enable it to tan more easily when you start exposing it to the sun. Remember to pack a large bottle of moisturizer or after-sun lotion to take on holiday and use after each sunbathing session. Always apply as much as the body will absorb, to keep the skin moist at all times and help prevent it from peeling.

Skin types vary considerably from one individual to another and it is very important to recognize fully which category you fall into. Almost all skin types contain melanin. This substance is stimulated by the sun's ultra-violet rays and combines with the haemoglobin in our blood to develop a tan. The depth of tan varies from person to person because of the varying amounts of melanin each individual's body produces. In most people melanin is distributed evenly throughout the body, resulting in an even tan. However, various degrees of care are needed to achieve this. Those with an oily skin are likely to tan easily and rarely burn, whilst those with fair, sensitive or freckled skin have a much greater risk of burning. Whatever your skin type, it is essential that you take adequate steps to protect it from the harmful rays of the sun.

It usually takes about three days for the melanin to reach the surface and help develop a proper tan. It is during these first three days that you must exercise extreme caution, patience and common sense. Many people burn on the first day of their holiday because they do not realize the strength of the sun's rays. Always make sure you choose a sunscreen with a protection factor to suit your skin type. In general, the higher the factor, the greater the protection. Personally, I have found it worthwhile to have a variety of factor creams. A high one for the first few days that my skin is exposed to the sun, a middle one for the next two or three days and then, as the tan develops, I switch to a lower factor cream to help gently build the tan that is now established. However, children and those with fair or sensitive skins should always use a high-factor protection sunscreen.

High-factor protection sunscreens should also be used on the areas not exposed to everyday sunlight such as: upper legs, back, chest and shoulders. In particular, don't forget to apply protection cream to the neck, as this is always exposed. Also, when applying sunscreen, care must be taken not to overlook the sides of our body and, typically, the small area just above our shorts and just below the legs of the shorts. In our anxiety not to get cream on the fabric, we often overlook these crucial areas, which can result in some very sore patches. Noses are a particular magnet for the sun and should be given extra protection. Apply sunscreen twenty minutes before you go out into the sun to allow the skin to absorb it, and reapply at least every two hours and after swimming. If you are a keen swimmer or water-sports fan it is a good idea to invest in a water-resistant sunscreen.

Wear a wide-brimmed hat to protect the top of your head, your nose, lips and neck. Many people also suffer from cold sores on their lips as a result of exposure to extreme sunlight. Make sure you have a creamy lipstick or a lip salve stick to apply before you go out into the sun.

Always be aware of the hidden strength of the sun. For example, at high altitudes the air is thinner and the sun stronger. Also, a breeze can make a really strong sun seem deceptively cooler. Remember, sunscreens are not just for sunbathing. Use them even when walking, sightseeing or eating out of doors.

In order to minimize the risks to our health it is extremely important not to overdo our suntanning campaign. Sensible, gentle tanning will lessen the risk, but those who fry in the Mediterranean sunshine for two weeks a year are just asking for trouble. Not only are they risking their health, but they will cause their skin to age prematurely. This is caused by the fibrous tissue just under the surface of the skin losing its elasticity which results in wrinkles and coarse sallow skin. To prevent premature ageing of the face apply a complete sunblock. You can always follow this with an artificial suntanning cream if you wish.

Build up your tan slowly, avoiding the midday sun. Sunbathe only in the early morning or late afternoon when the sun's rays are less fierce. Acclimatize your body to the sun by exposing it for just ten minutes on the first day and increasing gradually. Never stay in the sun till your skin goes red – the damage will have already been done. Remember, sunburn and sunstroke are painful and dangerous.

TEN TIPS FOR SUNCARE SENSE

1. Always choose a sunscreen with a protection factor to suit your skin type. Remember, the higher the factor the greater the degree of protection.

2. Young children and people with fair or sensitive skins should always use a sunscreen with a high-protection factor.

3. Try out your sunscreen lotions on the whole family *before* you go away in case one of you has an allergic reaction.

4. Apply sunscreens twenty minutes before you go out into the sun and reapply at least every two hours and after swimming.

5. Protect your face from premature wrinkles and facial lines by using a complete sunblock.

6. Wear a wide-brimmed hat to protect your head, neck, ears, nose and lips.

7. Avoid sunbathing between the hours of 11 a.m. and 2 p.m. when the sun's rays are at their fiercest.

8. Always be aware of the hidden strength of the sun and make sure you use adequate protection even on cloudy days.

9. Take plenty of moisturizing or after-sun lotion away with you and apply each evening to prevent the skin from drying out or peeling.

10. Never let your skin burn. Remember, a tan acquired slowly will last longer.

Skin Care and Make-up

Some women are fortunate enough to look delightful without make-up. Regrettably, I am not among them. I therefore felt it was important to include some basic tips and hints.

Personally, I use a combination of products ranging from a high street chemist's own brand to some more expensive ones. I select the products I use because I find them easy to apply and they suit my sensitive skin.

1. For your daily routine, you should choose products designed to suit your personal skin type be it normal, oily, dry, extra-dry, sensitive or a combination.

2. Always cleanse, tone and moisturize morning and night.

3. Remember 'we are what we eat' so a healthy balanced diet is an important part of our beauty routine.

Foundation creams

1. Always choose a shade which matches your own skin tone and test (ideally on the inner part of your arm) before making your final choice.

2. Before applying foundation, always make sure your skin is clean and moisturized.

3. Use a concealer to cover any spots, blemishes or under-eye shadows, before applying foundation.

4. Using fingertips or a damp cosmetic sponge, quickly and gently smooth the foundation over your face. Begin in the centre, blending carefully outwards to your hairline and down to the base of your neck.

5. Finally, pat pressed or loose powder over your face and neck and dust off any excess powder using a large, soft-bristle brush.

Blushers

1. For a natural finish and perfect colour blending always apply cream blusher *under* complexion powder and powder blush *over* complexion powder.

2. Apply a little colour at a time, blending from the fullest part of the cheeks towards the temples for a perfect blush look.

3. To light up the complexion and add emphasis, apply a touch of blush to the tip of the chin and on either side of the forehead close to the hairline.

4. Choose shades that complement your lipstick and eye shadow tones. Blusher should be applied after your lipstick to achieve the most accurate balance.

5. For evenings use a little extra blusher. Artificial lights can give the skin a 'washed out' look.

Eyes

1. When choosing eye shadows remember dark tones add depth and serve to 'diminish', while light tones accentuate and highlight.

2. Always apply mascara using upward strokes to top and underside of upper lashes and side strokes to lower lashes. Allow lashes to dry in between coats to prevent clogging.

3. Use an old toothbrush to brush eyebrows into a sleek shape and to blend in your make-up base with the hair-line edges.

Lips

1. Enhance the shape of your lips by tracing a contour line along your natural lip line with a lip pencil. Apply lipstick and then blot with a tissue. Re-apply for a long-lasting lip colour.

2. Use light colour shades to make the lips look fuller and dark shades to make the lips look thinner.

3. To make teeth look pearly white, use darker shades of lipstick and avoid pale pink shades if teeth are naturally ivory.

4. Change your toothbrush regularly and use dental floss every day. It is so worthwhile and important to look after your teeth properly.

Hair Care in the Sunshine

While we may like the fact that the colour of our hair gets lighter during the summer months, if it is exposed to excessive sun, sea and chlorine it can suffer quite dramatically.

To some degree, our hair benefits from the vitamins that we obtain from the sun and which help to give it a glossy, healthy shine. However, unlike our skin, which we can feel when it is burning, our hair has no feeling and we are therefore less likely to take steps to protect it. Just as our skin can become dried out through exposure to excessive sunlight, so too can our hair, leaving it brittle and prone to breakage. We should, therefore, take the time and trouble to prepare our hair for the sunlight, just as we do our skin.

Our aim should be to get our hair into as good a condition as possible well before we start exposing it to the summer sun. Hair is likely to be far more resilient if it is in good shape and a visit to a professional hairdresser to assess the condition of your hair and to receive the appropriate advice as to the best product to protect it is a wise course of action.

I speak from personal experience, for using a shampoo and conditioner designed to protect my hair through the summer months has proved extremely worthwhile.

A month before you are due to go on holiday step up your conditioning routine – and if you benefit from having a perm, make sure that this is done at least three weeks prior to your departure. This will give it time to settle down and give you the chance to get accustomed to handling it.

You may choose to use a semi-permanent colouring to enhance your hair in the summer. Most semi-permanent colours have a deep conditioning effect which can greatly benefit the condition of the hair as well as enriching the colour. For instance, a long-lasting cosmetic colouring can last up to twelve washes without you having any worries of re-growth. Lighter coloured hair can be made to look even lighter by having highlights put in. This should be done a little nearer to the time of departure.

If you swim a lot then obviously a short style is going to be infinitely more convenient. However, medium-length hair can be pinned up with a butterfly clip, which makes the hair easy to care for and at the same time gives it a sophisticated appearance during the day. Never use elastic bands around your hair, always use a clip, or a protected band – there are lots to choose from. Remember to use mousses, gels, creams and sprays that can transform an everyday style into something more exciting and also offer additional protection in the sun.

For those with hair in good condition and who want to keep it that way, the best advice is to wear a hat in the sun. This is especially important for children and also for men who are thinning on top – a sunburnt scalp can be very painful. For those who do not wish to wear a hat, there are products available that offer sunscreen for the hair.

Chlorine and sea-salt are enemies to the hair as well – they cause depletion of its natural oils and leave it brittle. Chlorine may discolour naturally fair hair and distort the colour of tinted or bleached hair, so hair should be rinsed and preferably shampooed after each swimming session. Hair will not be damaged from such frequent washing providing a good shampoo and conditioner is used every time.

Don't be a slave to your hair on holiday, but with some careful planning and preparation your hair can be one of your best beauty assets.

TEN TIPS FOR HEALTHY HOLIDAY HAIR

1. While away, keep your hairstyle simple and dress it up by using scarves, scrunches, combs and hairbands.

2. Look out for mini-sizes of your favourite products to save valuable packing space.

3. Keep a non-aerosol hairspray in your hand luggage to pep up your style while travelling.

4. Never brush wet hair – it is at its most fragile in this state and can easily stretch or break. Use a wide-toothed comb instead.

5. Wear long hair in a French plait during the day – this not only keeps tangles at bay and looks stylish, but when you let it down you'll be left with rippling waves.

6. Switch to a moisturizing shampoo and condition your hair after every wash.

7. Take a spray-on conditioner which can be combed through your hair when you're on the beach to give extra protection and to minimize tangles.

8. Avoid the application of suntan lotions around the hairline as they can cause a greasy build-up. Tinted lotions can also discolour roots.

9. Limit the use of heated appliances – it is preferable to towel-dry hair gently and then let it dry naturally instead.

10. Book your post-holiday hair trim appointment before you leave.

Hair Removal

As the summer approaches, one of the most important tasks is to remove any unwanted body hair. There are various methods available, of which shaving is still the most popular. However, re-growth is always rapid and because the ends of the hair have been made blunt when shaved, it tends to make the hairs appear thicker and more stubbly. While shaving under the arms is totally acceptable, I would never recommend shaving legs. Hair-removal creams and lotions are a better alternative if they will work for you. Regrettably, some women have such strong hair that such creams have little effect. These depilatory products work by dissolving the keratin (protein) from which the hair is made, from within the follicle, just below the surface of the skin. This leaves the skin feeling smooth and stubble-free and re-growth takes between 2 to 3 weeks. The benefit of these products is that they are painless and relatively convenient to use at home.

For those who find such products ineffective or wish for a longer-lasting result, waxing has to be the best option. It is one of the most effective ways of getting rid of unwanted hair as the hair is removed from the root and, therefore, re-growth takes much longer (up to 6 weeks). The hair becomes finer and less obvious after continuous waxing. Waxing can be done professionally or at home by using strip wax. Various packs are on sale at your local chemist, prepared in different-sized strips and differing strengths for different parts of the body. Although this method of hair removal is very effective, it can also be quite painful. It really depends on your pain threshold! Having our legs waxed professionally produces the best results, but it is more expensive.

Whether using a depilatory cream or strip wax, it is essential that the instructions are read carefully and fully before trying out the product.

One final warning. If you are planning to use an artificial suntan lotion prior to your holiday, ensure that you remove your unwanted body hair before application, particularly if using a depilatory cream. Otherwise you will find that the cream removes the effect of your tanning lotion.

Summer Nail Care

Finding time to give ourselves a manicure is always a problem, but in the summer months we really need to make time to paint our nails so that we can add some colour to our body when it is more exposed. In all probability we will be wearing fewer clothes, so jewellery, nail varnish and lipstick have a real role to play. In addition, wearing nail varnish is actually good for our nails. It protects them and gives them extra strength. Also, when we've painted our nails we are more likely to treat them with greater respect – for example, wearing rubber gloves when doing the washing-up or gardening.

There are many ways even the busiest people can have beautiful nails. Hand creams are important, and regular application of moisturizing cream, well rubbed in to the cuticles, can keep the skin soft and well cared for. Also, use a cuticle cream whenever you have time in order to keep the half-moons showing and looking healthy. Applying nail varnish need not take hours. I always put on a base coat before the application of a coloured nail enamel. This helps to prevent discoloration of the natural nail. If you don't have a lot of time to allow your nails to dry naturally, there are products which can be sprayed on to encourage the nails to dry quickly. However, I have always found that the best time to paint one's nails is last thing at night when all the washing-up is done.

Unfortunately, if we have long nails, occasionally one will tear or break. There are products available such as 'quick-set nail repair glue' which can save the day. All you have to do is to apply a droplet of the glue on to the split. Working it in with the applicator, hold the split together with tweezers for 10 seconds. Allow a couple of minutes for the glue to set and the nail is quite secure. This product has saved the day for me on several occasions when I desperately wanted to have even-length nails!

Remember to remove any nail enamel after seven days and, ideally, leave the nails clear of varnish for one day a week. This allows the nails to breathe and will help to prevent discoloration.

While some people have found that the condition of their nails improved as a result of following my low-fat diet, some, including myself initially, experienced nails splitting. By keeping the nails regularly manicured and painted with nail enamel, the nails will soon return to their normal state. Now, some six years after I embarked on my low-fat diet, my nails have never been stronger.

4

Planning Your Packing

If we were allowed to take an unlimited number of suit-cases on holiday with us, we could be less careful about the amount we pack, but with any holidays that involve flying, we are restricted by the weight allowance. The key to economical packing is careful planning. Before purchasing new items for your holiday, carefully examine clothes that are already in your wardrobe. Try to establish a couple of colour schemes so that you are not taking six pairs of shoes and six different handbags. A carefully colour-coordinated holiday wardrobe can be used to maximum effect, but only takes minimum space.

Anticipate your likely holiday programme and pack accordingly. Divide your clothes into sections – for the beach, sightseeing and evening. Take time to think it through and only pack the clothes that you are sure you will wear. Having made your final selection, check through it again and see which items you could leave behind. I have not yet met anyone who has not taken enough to wear on holiday – we are usually guilty of taking far too much.

I hope you will find the following advice helpful for your holiday this year.

TEN TIPS FOR PERFECT PACKING

1. Save partly used cosmetics, shampoos, conditioners and medication creams for when you go away. They weigh less and can save on valuable weight allowance.

2. Pack underwear into shoes to save space and prevent unnecessary squashing.

3. Place heavier and odd-shaped items (such as shoes or handbags) at the bottom of the case and fill in the gaps with swimwear, belts, socks, etc. Lay clothes on top, folding them as little as possible.

4. Place cosmetics, hairsprays and shampoos in a separate small bag that is waterproof, in case they break or leak.

5. Plan your holiday wardrobe carefully and adopt a colour scheme to coordinate with your shoes and handbags. Hang your clothes in 'outfits' so that unnecessary items can be left behind.

6. Roll up belts to prevent damaging them but pack ties by folding them in half and laying them flat.

7. Pack handkerchiefs in one handbag and jewellery in another.

8. Pack shoes in plastic bags to prevent any polish etc. from discolouring clothes and place a layer of tissue paper (not newspaper) or an old dry-cleaning bag between clothes to prevent creasing.

9. Take a large plastic bag in which soiled clothes can be stored.

10. If flying, weigh your suitcase *before* you leave, to check that you have not exceeded your weight allowance. Details of the weight allowance will be on your air ticket.

Holiday First-Aid kit

Don't let your holiday be ruined by illness. By following these simple guidelines and taking a limited number of medicated items with you, you may be able to save you and your family a great deal of anxiety and discomfort.

If you are taking any prescribed drugs be sure to take an adequate supply with you, and write on a separate piece of paper, which you keep with you, the names of all the drugs together with their strength. Should you be away from your hotel or separated from your luggage, such information could be invaluable in case of an emergency or accident.

While we don't want to fill our suitcase with unnecessary medication, I think the following items are worth taking:

Alka-Seltzer, plus anti-diarrhoea medicine.
Paracetamol.
Antiseptic cream.
Insect repellent.
Anti-histamine cream and tablets – for insect bites.
Crepe bandage with safety pin.
Variety pack of plasters.
Pair of small scissors.
Tweezers.
Antibiotics – if you are likely to be away for some time in a
     remote area.
Calamine lotion.
Thermometer – especially if taking children.
Water-purifying tablets – or drink only bottled water.
Personally prescribed medicines.
Travel-sickness tablets.

If you are travelling abroad, check with your doctor to see if any vaccinations are necessary. Sometimes these need to be done up to six weeks prior to departure, so plan well ahead.

5

Security – Home and Abroad

There can be nothing worse after being away on a well-earned holiday than to return to a house that has been burgled in your absence. Similarly, if you are away from home and personal items are stolen or lost, a holiday can be spoiled unless preventive action has been taken.

Below, I give some advice on security based on my own experience of travelling the world promoting my books. Taking a little time and trouble prior to departure can save weeks of misery that may follow.

TEN TIPS FOR A SECURE HOLIDAY

1. It is imperative when travelling abroad to take out adequate insurance, not only to cover your personal possessions and luggage, but also to cover medical expenses and every possible eventuality that may occur.

2. Before you leave, make two photocopies of your passport, flight tickets, credit cards and driving licence. Keep one copy of each at home and the other somewhere with you but separate from the original documents. If you should be unfortunate enough to lose them or have them stolen, you'll have all the information to hand and should be able to get replacements quickly.

3. Always label your luggage clearly with your flight number and destination. Use the labels issued by your travel agent. Luggage also needs to be labelled in case it gets lost in transit, but displaying your home address is unwise when travelling – you never know who's reading it! Instead, write your name and telephone number on a card and put it inside your luggage, or buy a concealed luggage label which will keep your address hidden from prying eyes.

4. Many suitcases look alike. To spot yours easily and quickly, tie a piece of coloured string or elastic band to the handle. It can save you from any embarrassing confusion.

5. Do tell the airport staff if you are carrying anything electrical in your luggage. You may be asked to dismantle electrical items kept in your hand luggage or to play them – so, for example, keep a tape handy to play on your personal stereo.

6. After a long holiday you may forget where you have left your car-park ticket or even whereabouts in the car park you have left your car. Keep your ticket somewhere safe and note on the back of it the floor level etc. where you parked your car. Also, remember to retain enough money to pay for the car parking, taxi, bus or train fare home.

7. In case your flight is delayed, keep in your hand luggage some basic toiletries (make-up, deodorant, hairspray, toothbrush and toothpaste) and something to read or do. Also ensure that you have enough money to buy refreshments, in case your delay turns out to be a long one.

8. Make sure you have a contact name from your travel agent, or someone who is available after hours, should you experience any problems.

9. Tell your neighbours if you are going away and ask them to keep an eye on your home during your holiday. Don't forget to cancel your milk and papers. It is also possible for the Post Office to hold on to your mail in your absence.

10. Automatic time switches which will turn your house lights on and off will certainly help to give the impression someone is at home while you are away. Security locks on doors and windows are always a good investment too.

PART II

Waistline Survival
On Holiday

6

Holidaying in Hotels

The variety and quality of food served in hotels can vary as much as the hotels themselves, but most establishments are very helpful in providing for any specific dietary needs, particularly if you explain that they are health-related.

The key to avoiding weight gain on holiday is to take an overall view of your eating plan for the day. If you know you'll be sitting down to a three- or four-course dinner each evening, then try to have light meals at breakfast and lunch.

Depending on the type of hotel, the choice of menu will vary enormously. As a simple guide, select your starter with care, avoiding anything obviously high in fat. For the main course, fish and chicken dishes are the best choices for low-fat dining, but check before ordering that the recipe doesn't involve deep-frying or pastry. Ask (if possible) for the vegetables (and everything else) to be served without butter. For dessert, avoid those dishes that are cake- and pastry-based and say 'no' to cream. Fruit served in wine or liqueur is fine and can actually be more tasty without cream. The cheeseboard should be avoided. Always order sparkling mineral water to help space out the consumption of alcoholic drinks – these should be drunk in moderation, particularly when on a sun-based holiday.

Dieters should aim to select from the following **Green List** whenever possible and non-dieters are recommended to follow the suggestions in the **Amber List**, with only the occasional indulgence from the **Red List**!

GREEN LIST

Starters:

- Grapefruit
- Sorbet
- Melon
- Consommé or any clear soup
- Bread roll
- Mixed salad with oil-free dressing
- Smoked trout
- Corn on the cob – without butter

AMBER LIST

Starters:

- Smoked mackerel
- Rollmop herring
- Regular soups
- Smoked salmon
- Mixed hors d'oeuvres
- Prawn cocktail
- Parma ham and melon
- Corn on the cob – with butter
(most of the butter falls off!)

RED LIST

Starters:

- Whitebait
- Salami
- Cream soups
- Avocado pear
- Garlic prawns
- Regular spaghetti bolognese
- Pasta, cooked in butter or with cream
- Cheese dishes
- Garlic bread

GREEN LIST

Main courses:

- Chicken or fish dishes, cooked without fat
- Lean steak, grilled
- Pork steak, grilled
- Potatoes, cooked without fat
- Rice, boiled
- Pasta, served without butter or cream
- Turkey
- Liver, not fried
- Roast meat, with all fat removed
- Trout, not fried
- Any vegetables, cooked without fat
- Gammon, grilled, with all fat removed
- Prawns, cooked without butter or oil

AMBER LIST

Main courses:

- Chicken or fish in cream sauce
- Casserole dishes
- Any meat served in sauce
- Regular spaghetti bolognese
- Roast potatoes
- Chips (thick-cut)
- Vegetables served in butter

RED LIST

Main courses:

- Chicken in breadcrumbs, deep-fried
- Chicken Kiev
- Fish and chips
- Any fish in batter or breadcrumbs, deep-fried
- Any meat pies
- Chips (thin-cut)

GREEN LIST

Desserts:

- Oranges in Cointreau
- Pears in meringue
- Fresh fruit salad
- Pears in red wine
- Fresh pineapple in Kirsch
- Sorbet
- Fresh fruit
- Coffee with milk

AMBER LIST

Desserts:

- Crème caramel
- Trifle
- Pavlova
- Ice cream
- Fruit-based mousse

RED LIST

Desserts:

- Gateau
- Pies
- Tarts
- Cheesecake
- Shortbread
- Sponge puddings
- Cheese and biscuits
- Chocolate mousse or soufflé
- Roulade
- Cream
- Chocolates
- Coffee with cream

7

Maximizing on Bed and Breakfast

Whether it's a spare room in a private house, an average size guesthouse, or a large hotel, we can be certain that if we have booked for bed and breakfast, the breakfast will be substantial – especially in England and northern Europe. In fact, I think the smaller establishments serve by far the largest breakfasts.

Whatever the environment, it is perfectly reasonable for a guest to want the best value for money. I so often hear from my holiday-making dieters – 'Well, I paid for it so I was jolly well going to eat it!' And I'm not going to argue with that dictum because it is a sound one. But I *will* endeavour, in the following pages, to steer you in the direction of a hearty, healthy and low-fat breakfast.

I would never expect anyone actually to lose weight on holiday, so I am not suggesting that you should stick to any particular diet. However, by selecting carefully from the categories of breakfast food listed in this chapter, it is possible to maintain your weight. Another factor to bear in mind is that we are often more physically active when we are away from home. Moreover, it is also important to consider what you are likely to be eating at lunch time. If you are planning a light lunch, perhaps just fruit, obviously you can justify a good feast at breakfast time! But remember, calories *do* count and if we overeat even low-fat foods, we *can* gain weight.

Finally, to derive maximum enjoyment from the food that is offered to you, it is well worth having a chat with the cook or chef to ask if they can prepare your food without fat – 'for health reasons'. They are usually most anxious to oblige and it will give you greater freedom.

The Holiday-Maker's Guide to Breakfasts

Remember that the **Green List** offers foods that are either fat-free or very low in fat. Dieters may select freely, but in moderation, from this list.

The **Amber List** contains foods which are either a little higher in fat content or high in calories because of their high sugar content e.g. dried fruit. Non-dieters may select freely from either the **Green** or **Amber Lists** for a healthy and nutritious menu.

The **Red List** itemizes those foods that are very high in fat. These foods should be strictly avoided by dieters and in any case they are significantly less healthy than those foods listed in the **Green** and **Amber Lists**. Non-dieters should, therefore, still restrict their consumption to an absolute minimum for the benefit of their health.

GREEN LIST

Continental-type breakfasts:
(select freely)

- Semi-skimmed milk (if possible)
- Cereal
- Porridge
- Honey
- Grapefruit or other tinned fruit
- Stewed fruit
- Fresh fruit
- Yogurt – diet brands
- Toast, bread, rolls etc.
- Jam, marmalades
- Preserves

Cooked breakfasts:

- Tomatoes, not fried
- Mushrooms, not fried
- Bacon, grilled, with all fat removed
- Toast
- Baked beans

AMBER LIST

Continental-type breakfasts:
(select in moderation)

- Green figs and dates
- Dried fruit
- Sugar
- Greek yogurt
- Non-diet brands of yogurt
- Low-fat spreads containing less than 30% fat (i.e. 30 g of fat per 100 g)
- Croissants (eaten without butter or margarine)

Cooked breakfasts:

- Kippers, cooked without butter
- Sausages, grilled
- Eggs, poached or boiled
- Eggs, scrambled without butter

RED LIST

Continental-type breakfasts:
(select sparingly)

- Croissants, spread with butter or margarine
- Danish pastries
- Butter, margarine (containing more than 30% fat) or low-fat spreads or margarines low in cholesterol or high in polyunsaturates
- Salamis and pâtés

Cooked breakfasts:

- Fried eggs
- Fried bread
- Fried sausages
- Fried bacon
- Fried black pudding
- Scrambled eggs, cooked with butter
- Kippers, cooked with butter

8

Surviving Self-Catering

We choose self-catering holidays for a variety of reasons. It may be that we prefer the freedom of doing our own thing and not having to toe the line within the rules and regulations laid down by a hotel, or perhaps we like the challenge of discovering the local foods in unfamiliar shops and markets and having fun preparing them. Some find self-catering a more economical option if they have a large family. However, I see one enormous advantage in opting for self-catering. If we cook our own food we are in total control of what we eat and how it is prepared. And, of course, there is always the possibility of dining out if we want a treat.

If you decide to go self-catering, discuss with the family in advance what the action plan will be. Breakfast is simple to organize with fruit juice, cereal, toast and marmalade for a quick option, but if you prefer a late start you can have a more substantial 'brunch' instead – perhaps cereal, followed by grilled bacon, tomatoes, mushrooms, baked beans, with toast and marmalade to finish. Such a meal should keep you going until the evening, with, maybe, a small ice cream or piece of fruit at 3 p.m. to sustain you through the afternoon.

TEN TIPS FOR SELF-CATERING

1. Cook without fat at all times. (Buy a non-stick spray for the frying pan if necessary.)
2. Try fresh local breads and rolls, but do not use butter, margarine or even low-fat spreads. Instead, use reduced-oil salad dressing, mustard or pickles.
3. Buy local, lean, cooked meats and salad to fill rolls and sandwiches for beach lunches, and locally caught fish for your evening meal.
4. Don't buy biscuits or cakes; try the unusual locally grown fruits instead.
5. Drink low-calorie soft and fizzy drinks in place of high-sugar ones.
6. Don't prepare more food than you think you'll need. In hot climates, leftovers won't keep and you might be tempted to eat them up rather than throw food away.
7. Plan your menus ahead and only buy what you actually need.
8. Pack a small roll of clingfilm so that packed lunches can be parcelled up for each individual – it avoids temptation for dieters.
9. Dieters should try to eat food similar to that of the rest of the family. Even the odd ice cream is permissible, but if you want a big one, have it as a lunch!
10. Try to be as physically active as possible. Disco-dancing is a great way to work off those pounds (kg)!

9

Five-Minute Beach Workout

Spending hours lying in the glorious sunshine needn't be as idle as it looks. Here are some simple ideas to help you discreetly keep in shape while you tan. The usual warm-up routine is not necessary in this context as your body will be thoroughly warm from lying in the hot sun.

1. Sitting up with your hands supporting you on either side, cross your ankles and, keeping your legs straight, attempt to separate them by pushing the ankles together. Hold the extreme position for 2 counts, then relax. Repeat 5 times, then change over ankles and repeat. (Good for outer thighs.)

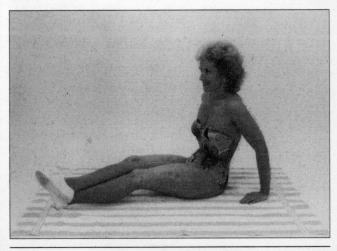

2. Bend your knees and place your hands as far behind you as possible with your fingers pointing forwards. Bending your arms, lower your upper body backwards towards the ground and straighten them again without locking the elbows. Repeat as many times as possible without discomfort.

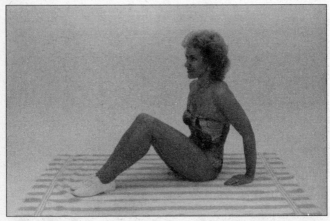

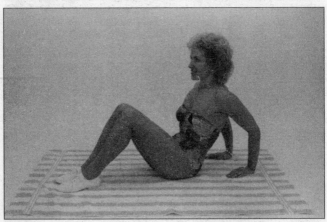

NB: Elbows should bend backwards, not outwards. (This is good for the under-arm area.)

3. Prop yourself up on your elbows and place a beach ball between your knees. Squeeze the ball as many times as possible with your knees and inner thighs. (This is good for the inner thigh area.

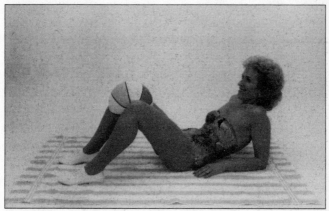

4. Lying on your side, propped up on one arm and with the lower leg bent, raise and lower the other leg and at the same time press down on it with the ball. This added resistance works the outer thigh muscles harder and is therefore even more effective. Roll over and repeat on the other side.

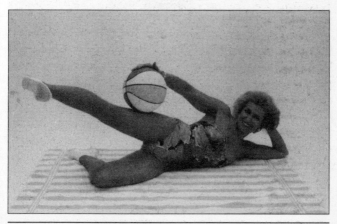

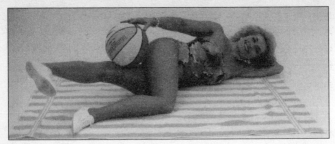

5. Lying on your side, head resting on one arm, bend the
top leg and rest it on the ground in front of you. Place the
beach ball on to the inner thigh of your lower leg and hold
it firmly with your free hand. Raise and lower the straight
lower leg, pressing the ball firmly against it to increase
resistance. Repeat as many times as you can without discomfort. Roll over and repeat with the other leg. (This
exercise works the inner thighs.)

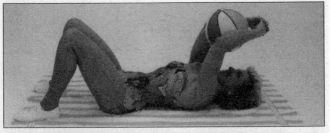

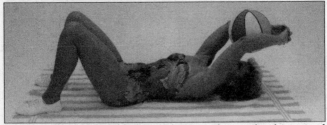

6. Lie down with your knees bent and your back pressed
flat against the ground. Place the beach ball between your
elbows and squeeze them together. As you squeeze, push

your arms backwards over your head. Slowly bend the arms forwards to the starting position and repeat the backwards and forwards movement as many times as is comfortable. (This exercise works the muscles in the chest and arms.)

7. Sitting propped up by your arms, place the ball between your bent knees. Simultaneously squeeze your knees together and dip down, with your bent elbows behind you, as many times as you can comfortably. (This works the inner thighs and the backs of the arms simultaneously.)

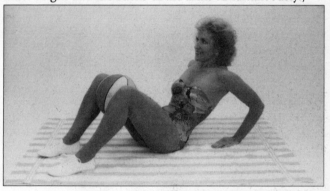

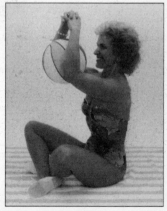

8. Sitting up cross-legged, place the beach ball between your elbows at shoulder level and squeeze 20 times. (This exercise works the muscles across the chest.)

9. Sitting cross-legged, place a towel behind your neck and hold it taut at each end. Sitting as straight as possible, slowly raise the towel behind your head and as high as possible, then lower it again to the starting position. Repeat the exercise as many times as is comfortable. (This works the shoulders and upper back and is particularly helpful in improving posture.)

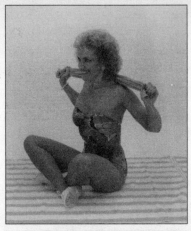

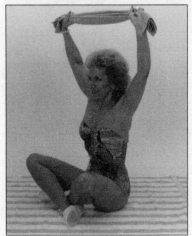

PART III

Summer At Home

10

3-Day Post-Holiday Corrector Diet

No matter how much self-control you have exercised while on holiday, most people inevitably come home having gained a few pounds (kg) of 'excess baggage'! With this in mind, I have devised a quick 'repair package' to enable you to return to your pre-holiday shape with the minimum of effort. Start this post-holiday corrector diet as soon as you can on your return but do not follow it for more than three days.

Daily Allowance:

5 fl oz (125 ml) unsweetened fruit juice
10 fl oz (250 ml) skimmed or semi-skimmed milk

DAY 1

Breakfast

1 oz (25 g) All-Bran with 4 oz (100 g) sliced strawberries, and milk from allowance.

Lunch

6 oz (150 g) cottage cheese served with mixed salad.

Dinner

6 oz (150 g) grilled chicken (no skin) served with 4 oz (100 g) new potatoes and green vegetables, plus 1 piece fresh fruit.

DAY 2

Breakfast

1 oz (25 g) muesli, plus 5 oz (125 g) diet yogurt.

Lunch

1 lb (400 g) fresh fruit.

Dinner

8 oz (200 g) fish, steamed, grilled or microwaved and
served with unlimited vegetables and 4 oz (100 g)
new potatoes, plus 1 piece fresh fruit.

DAY 3

Breakfast

1/2 a melon, plus 1 tablespoon diet yogurt

Lunch

4 Ryvitas spread with Marmite and topped with
3 oz (75 g) cottage cheese.

Dinner

Vegetable Bake (*see recipe*) served with mixed fresh
vegetables, plus 1 diet yogurt.

11

Perfect Picnics

A picnic on a warm and sunny day can be fun to prepare and a delight to eat. If the whole family gets involved in the planning of such an outing it is almost certain to be a success. Whether it's lunch, tea or just a snack, you can still eat healthily and there is no need to abandon the diet if you've worked hard to shed a few pounds (kg) for the summer months. Try to make your family picnic an energetic time too. Don't forget the cricket bat and ball, the dog's lead and some suitable shoes!

Picnics should contain lots of different foods in order to cater for everyone's taste and it's quite easy to make them healthy as well as appetizing.

Make up your picnic menu from the ingredients listed below or see my suggestions for **Exciting Fillings for Summer Sandwiches** on page 221.

The foods itemized in the **Green List** are ideal for those on a reducing diet, whilst the **Amber List** offers healthy alternatives for non-dieters. Consumption of foods from the **Red List** should be kept to a minimum.

GREEN LIST

Bread or biscuits:

- Bread (no butter or spread)
- Ryvita

Sandwich fillings or salad ingredients:

- Chicken (no skin)
- Turkey
- Lean ham
- Lean beef
- Tuna (in brine)
- Cottage cheese
- Savoury Meat Loaf (*see recipe*)
- Low-calorie coleslaw
- Marmite
- All salad vegetables
- Asparagus
- Salmon (in moderation)
- Mackerel (in moderation)
- Prawns
- Crab

Dressings and spreads:

- Any fat-free dressing
- Reduced-oil salad dressing (any brand) in moderation
- Branston pickle
- Mustard
- Brown sauce, etc.

Snack items:

- Pickles
- Vegetables sticks with a low-fat dip

Cakes and desserts:

- Cakes made without fat
- Fresh fruit
- Low-fat yogurts
- Low-fat fromage frais
- Meringues
- Jelly-type desserts
- Banana and Sultana cake (*see recipe*)

Drinks:

- Tea and coffee with low-fat milk
- Low-calorie drinks
- 1 glass wine
- Unsweetened fruit juice

AMBER LIST

Bread or biscuits:

- Bread spread with low-fat spread
- Water biscuits
- Any crispbreads

Sandwich fillings or salad ingredients:

- Eggs
- Low-fat cheddar
- Edam
- Low-fat soft cheese
- Salmon
- Mackerel
- Chicken liver pâté
- Tongue
- Corned beef
- Low-fat sausages, grilled

Dressings and spreads:

- Low-calorie dressings or mayonnaise

Snack items:

- Twiglets
- Low-fat crisps
- Low-fat snacks

Cakes and desserts:

- Jaffa cakes
- Ice cream (not Cornish)
- Low-calorie desserts
- Dried fruit
- Regular yogurts or creamy varieties

Drinks:

- Tea and coffee with full-fat milk
- Regular fizzy drinks
- Yogurt drinks
- Skimmed-milk drinks
- Alcoholic drinks

RED LIST

Bread or biscuits:

- Bread spread with butter or margarine
- Cream crackers and other savoury biscuits

Sandwich fillings or salad ingredients:

- Full-fat hard and soft cheeses
- Pâté (other than chicken liver pâté)
- Salami
- German sausage
- Sausages
- Pork pies
- Haslet
- Black pudding
- Scotch eggs
- Samosas
- Salads mixed with cream or mayonnaise
- Avocado
- Chicken fried in breadcrumbs

Dressings and spreads:

- Mayonnaise
- French dressing
- Any dressing made with oil or cream

Snack items:

- Full-fat crisps and snacks
- Peanuts
- Cheeselets and similar savoury biscuits
- Olives

Cakes and desserts:

- Other cakes, pastries and biscuits
- Cream
- Cornish ice cream
- Choc ice
- Crème brûlée

Drinks:

- Tea and coffee with cream
- Full-fat milk shakes
- Cream-based liqueurs

Exciting Fillings for Summer Sandwiches

Whenever possible choose wholemeal bread. Do not use butter or any other fat spread.

1. Spread each slice of bread with Marmite and fill with cottage cheese and grated carrot.

2. Spread each slice of bread with reduced-oil salad dressing (any brand) and fill with chopped or sliced cold chicken and sweetcorn.

3. *Triple-decker sandwiches*:

Using three slices of bread (preferably 2 brown and 1 white), spread the first slice with reduced-oil salad dressing (any brand), the second with mustard on one side and sweet pickle on the other, and the third slice with tomato ketchup.

Place mixed salad (lettuce, tomatoes, onion, cucumber) and 1 slice of chicken on top of the first slice of bread, place the second slice of bread on top with the pickle next to the chicken, and a slice of ham on top of the mustard-spread side, then cover with the remaining slice of bread spread with tomato sauce. Press down firmly, cut into triangles and pack each 'set' of triple sandwiches individually.

4. Mash one large banana and mix with 4 oz (100 g) low-fat cottage cheese. Spread straight on to the bread.

5. Make a prawn cocktail sauce by mixing 2 tablespoons of tomato ketchup with 3 tablespoons of reduced-oil salad dressing (any brand). Add a dash of Tabasco sauce if desired, then spread on to brown bread and fill with peeled prawns or crab.

6. Mix cottage cheese with reduced-oil salad dressing (any brand) and tinned salmon. Spread straight on to the bread and top with cucumber slices.

7. Spread one slice of bread with Marmite and another slice with reduced-oil salad dressing (any brand). Fill with cottage cheese and salad.

8. Spread one slice of bread with mustard and another slice with sweet pickle. Fill with sliced beef, turkey, ham or chicken and cold savoury stuffing (made with water only).

12

Barbecue Ideas

There's something rather special about a warm summer's evening and inviting a few friends over for a barbecue. And it is particularly satisfying to see the men doing the cooking and tending the charcoal. Here are a few tips for a happy and healthy barbecue:

1. Make sure you have enough charcoal, lighter fuel and matches before you start.

2. Keep a bucket of water handy in case of accidents. Also have a damp cloth, oven glove and towel to hand.

3. Prepare the meat by trimming off all the visible fat and allow it to marinate in a variety of spices mixed with a little wine for a few hours prior to cooking if possible.

4. Light the barbecue early and place scrubbed potatoes wrapped in tin foil on the racks as soon as the barbecue is lit.

5. Because we often eat barbecue food standing up, prepare lots of easy-to-eat salad dishes to serve with the meat, e.g. Carrot and Sultana Salad, Sweetcorn and Red Bean Salad (*see recipes*), low-calorie coleslaw, grated raw beetroot with sultanas, cherry tomatoes, shredded lettuce, cubed cucumber. (Also see **Light Lunches & Main Courses** and **Barbecue Specials** in the recipe chapter for further salad suggestions.)

6. Prepare a mix of low-fat plain yogurt, cottage cheese, Reduced-Oil Salad Dressing (*see recipe*) and sweetcorn to place on top of the potatoes instead of butter.

7. Keep the dessert simple. Fresh strawberries or raspberries are always popular. Serve with frozen yogurt or fromage frais.

8. Have sparkling mineral water available as well as wine.

9. Serve black grapes with the coffee.

10. Ask everyone to help take the plates and equipment inside. There's nothing worse than seeing last night's leftovers and unwashed crockery littering the garden the following morning.

Several of the recipes included in this book could be prepared for a barbecue. For a tasty selection of assorted kebabs and other dishes particularly suited to barbecuing, see **Barbecue Specials** in the recipe chapter.

13

Recipes

The recipes included in this chapter appear under the following headings:

LIGHT LUNCHES & MAIN COURSES
DESSERTS
BARBECUE SPECIALS
CAKES
DRESSINGS
DRINKS

Weights and measures

For convenience, the following conversion rates have been used throughout this recipe chapter:

$$
\begin{array}{rcl}
1 \text{ oz} & = & 25 \text{ g} \\
1 \text{ fl oz} & = & 25 \text{ ml} \\
1/2 \text{ pint} & = & 250 \text{ ml}
\end{array}
$$

LIGHT LUNCHES & MAIN COURSES

Carrot and Sultana Salad
(Serves 1)

2 large fresh carrots
1 oz (25 g) sultanas

Peel and grate the carrots, then mix with the sultanas. Serve with a green salad or on a jacket potato.

Cauliflower and Courgette Bake
(Serves 4)

2 onions
1 small to medium cauliflower
12 oz (300 g) courgettes
1 egg
2¹/2 oz (62.5 g) fromage frais or yogurt
2 teaspoons cornflour
¹/2 teaspoon French mustard
salt and pepper
4 oz (100 g) low-fat Cheddar cheese
1–2 oz (25–50 g) wholemeal breadcrumbs
2–3 teaspoons Parmesan cheese (optional)

Peel and slice the onions. Break the cauliflower into florets and thickly slice the courgettes.

Cook the onions in boiling salted water until they are almost tender. In another pan of boiling salted water, blanch the cauliflower florets for 5 minutes, then add the courgettes and cook for a further 2 minutes. Drain and chill under cold running water until the vegetables are cold. Drain well again and place in an oven-proof dish.

Beat the egg well and mix with the fromage frais or yogurt, cornflour and mustard. Season with salt and pepper. Beat well until smooth.

Dice the Cheddar cheese and add to the fromage frais mixture. Pour over the vegetables. Sprinkle the breadcrumbs over the top with the Parmesan cheese, if used.

Bake in a preheated oven at 190°C, 375°F, or Gas Mark 5, for about 25 minutes.

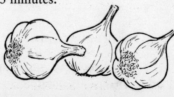

Chicken Curry
(Serves 2)

2 chicken joints
1 medium-sized onion
1 eating apple
15 oz (375 g) tinned tomatoes
1 bay leaf
2 teaspoons oil-free sweet pickle or Branston pickle
1 teaspoon tomato purée
1 tablespoon curry powder

Remove all fat and skin from the chicken joints. Chop the onion finely. Core the apple and chop into small pieces.

Place all the ingredients in a saucepan and bring to the boil. Cover and cook slowly for about 1 hour, stirring occasionally and turning the chicken joints every 15 minutes or so. If the mixture is too thin, remove the lid and cook on a slightly higher heat until the sauce reduces and thickens.

Serve on a bed of boiled brown rice (approximately 4 oz/100 g [cooked weight] per person).

Chicken and Mushroom Suprême
(Serves 4)

freshly ground black pepper
4 chicken breasts
soy sauce
8 oz (200 g) button mushrooms
2 teaspoons cornflour
6 tablespoons cold water

Preheat a non-stick frying pan and add a generous amount of freshly ground black pepper. Place the chicken in the hot pan and sprinkle more pepper on to the chicken. Sauté the chicken pieces until they have changed colour on all sides.

Cover with a lid, reduce the heat and continue to cook on a low heat for 20–30 minutes. Add more pepper at approximately 10-minute intervals, at the same time turning the chicken over.

When the chicken is almost cooked add 6 tablespoons soy sauce to the frying pan. Add the button mushrooms, cover and simmer for a further 10 minutes. Add more soy sauce as necessary to prevent the pan becoming too dry.

When the chicken and mushrooms are thoroughly cooked, place them on a preheated serving dish and keep warm.

Add more soy sauce to the frying pan until there is approximately ¼ pint (125 ml) fluid. Mix the cornflour and cold water together and carefully stir into the sauce in the pan. Remove from the heat as soon as it begins to thicken and stir vigorously to prevent it becoming lumpy. Return to the heat and cook gently for 2 or 3 minutes.

Serve with hot boiled rice (approximately 4 oz/100 g [cooked weight] brown rice per person). Place the rice in a preheated serving dish and put the chicken pieces and mushrooms in the centre. Pour the hot sauce over the chicken and mushrooms and serve immediately, with unlimited green vegetables.

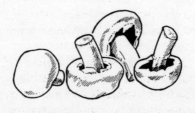

Chicken with Orange and Apricots
(Serves 4)

1 onion
2 large oranges
5 fl oz (125 ml) orange juice
5 fl oz (125 ml) dry white wine or cider
1 teaspoon arrowroot
4 chicken breasts or quarters
salt and pepper
8 oz (200 g) fresh apricots or
tinned apricots in natural juice
1 tablespoon chopped chervil or parsley

Peel the onion and chop finely. Peel the rind from 1 orange very thinly and cut into fine (julienne) strips. Blanch in a little boiling water for 4–5 minutes until tender. Drain but reserve the water. Reserve the strips of peel for garnishing. Cut away the pith from this orange and then cut out the orange segments. Grate the rind from the other orange and squeeze the juice.

Place the chopped onion in a pan with all the orange juice and the white wine or cider. Simmer gently until tender. Make the liquid up to 1/2 pint (250 ml) with the reserved liquid. Mix the arrowroot with a little water and add to the pan. Bring to the boil, stirring all the time.

Skin the chicken and place in an ovenproof casserole. Pour the sauce over and season to taste with salt and pepper. Cover and cook in a preheated oven at 180°C, 350°F, or Gas Mark 4, for about 30–35 minutes until the chicken is almost tender.

Halve the fresh apricots and remove the stones, or drain the tinned apricots. Add to the casserole and continue cooking for a further 10–20 minutes until the chicken and fruit are tender. Add the reserved orange segments about 5 minutes before the end of the cooking time so that they just heat through.

Check the seasoning. Pour into a hot dish or serve from the casserole. Sprinkle the strips of peel and the chervil or parsley over the top just before serving.

Chicken and Potato Pie
(Serves 4)

1 onion
1 lb (400 g) cooked chicken
1/2 pint (250 ml) skimmed milk
(in addition to allowance)
1 chicken stock cube
1 bay leaf
6 peppercorns
salt and freshly ground black pepper
1 dessertspoon cornflour
11/2 lbs (600 g) potatoes, peeled and cooked
21/2 oz (62.5 g) low-fat natural yogurt

Peel and slice the onion. Chop the chicken coarsely.

Place all but 2 fl oz (50 ml) of the skimmed milk in a non-stick saucepan with the onion, stock-cube, bay leaf and seasonings. Heat gently, then cover the pan. Simmer for 5 minutes to allow the flavours to infuse. Remove the peppercorns and bay leaf.

Mix the cornflour with the remaining cold milk and gradually add this to the saucepan and stir well. Slowly bring the sauce to the boil, stirring all the time. When boiling gently, add the chopped chicken. The sauce should be a thick creamy consistency. If is too thin the potato topping will sink. Add more slaked cornflour (i.e. mixed with milk) if necessary. Taste for seasoning and adjust as necessary.

Pour the chicken sauce into a pie dish, allowing space for the potato 'crust' to be added.

Mash the pre-cooked potatoes with the yogurt so that the mixture is creamy and light. Add more yogurt or skimmed milk as necessary. Season well. Carefully spoon the potato mixture on to the chicken sauce mixture, so that the dish is completely covered to the edges, and smooth over with a fork. Place the dish under a hot grill to brown the top. Serve immediately.

Alternatively, the pie can be made well in advance and then warmed through in a preheated moderate oven (180°C, 350°F, Gas Mark 4) for 20–30 minutes.

Chicken or Prawn Chop Suey
(Serves 4)

4 chicken joints or 12 oz (300 g) prawns
3 large carrots
5 sticks celery
6 oz (150 g) mange-tout (optional)
2 large onions
1 red pepper
2 green peppers
2 tins (30 oz/750 g) beansprouts or 1 pack of fresh
beansprouts
4 tablespoons vegetable stock
salt and pepper to taste
soy sauce

Prepare the ingredients as follows: skin, bone, then coarsely slice the chicken, or shell the prawns. Peel and coarsely grate the carrots. Finely chop the celery. Trim and wash the mange-tout, if using. Peel and finely slice the onions. Deseed all 3 peppers and slice them. Drain the tinned beansprouts.

Add the chicken to the vegetable stock and cook in a large non-stick frying pan or wok on a moderate heat until it changes colour. Add the carrots, celery, mange-tout and onions, and stir-fry. Add the sliced peppers and beansprouts and continue to cook until thoroughly hot, but do not overcook. Season to taste.

Serve on a bed of boiled brown rice, with soy sauce. Allow 4 oz (100 g) [cooked weight] rice per person.

Chicken Spaghetti
(Serves 4)

4 chicken breasts, skinned
freshly ground black pepper
1 large onion, finely chopped
2 cloves garlic, crushed
1 jar Dolmio or Ragu Bolognese Sauce
1 chicken stock cube
3 pints (1.7 litres) water
10 oz (250 g) spaghetti (non-egg variety)

Cut the chicken into bite-sized pieces with scissors or a sharp knife. Preheat a non-stick frying pan and add a generous amount of freshly ground black pepper. Place the chicken in the hot pan and dry-fry until it changes colour. Add the chopped onion and the crushed garlic and cook until the onion is soft. Stir in the Bolognese sauce and mix well. Cover the pan and continue cooking on a low heat for 15 minutes.

Meanwhile, dissolve the chicken stock cube in a large pan with 3 pints (1.7 litres) of water and bring to the boil. When the water is boiling add the spaghetti and cook according to the instructions on the packet; then drain it through a colander.

Serve on individual plates and place the chicken sauce in the centre, on top of the spaghetti.

Chinese Salad
(Serves 2)

8oz (200 g) fresh beansprouts
1 large carrot
½ Spanish onion
4 oz (100 g) cooked chicken breast
1 6 oz (150 g) tin mandarin oranges
in natural juice
2 oz (50 g) sultanas
1 tablespoon lemon juice
1 tablespoon soy sauce

Prepare the ingredients as follows: wash and drain the beansprouts; peel and coarsely grate the carrot; peel and finely slice the onion; skin, bone and chop the chicken into bite-sized cubes; drain the mandarin oranges and reserve the juice.

Mix together in a salad bowl the beansprouts, carrot, onion, chicken, mandarins and sultanas.

In a smaller bowl, add 2 tablespoons of the reserved juice from the mandarins to the lemon juice and soy sauce, and mix well. Sprinkle over the salad and toss well. Cover and keep chilled until ready to serve.

This salad must be eaten within 3 days of preparation.

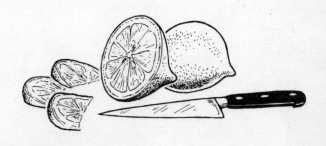

Coleslaw
(Serves 4)

2 large carrots
8 oz (200 g) white cabbage
1 Spanish onion
4 oz (100 g) Reduced-Oil Salad Dressing
(*see recipe*, page 280)

Wash the carrots and cabbage, then grate them; peel and finely chop the onion. Mix together in a bowl with the Reduced-Oil Salad Dressing.

Serve immediately or keep chilled and eat within 2 days.

Coq au Vin
(Serves 4)

3¹/₂–4 lbs (1.4–1.6 kg) roasting chicken
4 oz (100 g) back bacon, with all fat removed
4 oz (100 g) button onions
7 fl oz (175 ml) red wine (preferably Burgundy)
2 cloves garlic, crushed with ¹/₂ teaspoon salt
bouquet garni
¹/₄–¹/₂ pint (125–250 ml) chicken stock
salt and pepper
1 teaspoon cornflour
3 tablespoons water
chopped parsley, to garnish

Joint and skin the chicken and place in a non-stick frying pan. Over a fairly brisk heat, brown the chicken all over and then remove to one side while other ingredients are prepared. Cut the bacon into strips, approximately 1¹/₂ inches (3.75 cm) long, and blanch these and the onions by putting them in a pan of cold water, bringing to the boil and draining well.

Sauté the bacon and onions in the frying pan over a brisk heat until they are brown. Replace the chicken joints and pour over the wine. Bring to the boil and 'flame' by setting the pan alight with a match. This removes the alcohol from the wine.

Add the crushed garlic, bouquet garni, stock and seasoning. Cover the pan and cook slowly for about 1 hour, or place in a casserole and put in a preheated oven at 170°C, 325°F, or Gas Mark 3.

Test to see that the chicken is tender and that it is thoroughly cooked. Discard the bouquet garni, remove the chicken to one side and keep warm. Mix the cornflour and water to a smooth paste. Slowly pour this into the sauce, stirring continuously to keep it smooth. Return to the heat and boil, stirring all the time. Place the chicken pieces back into the casserole and pour the sauce over.

Garnish with parsley and serve immediately.

Fish Cakes
(Serves 4)

12 oz (300 g) potatoes
16 oz (400 g) cod
1 egg white
2 tablespoons fresh parsley, finely chopped
1 teaspoon prepared mustard
salt and freshly ground black pepper

Peel the potatoes and boil for 15–20 minutes until cooked. Meanwhile, bake, steam or microwave the cod until cooked. Remove any skin or bones from the fish and flake it. Drain the potatoes and mash until smooth. Mix the fish and the potatoes together. Add the egg white and stir well, then add the parsley, mustard, salt and pepper and mix again. Wet your hands and make fish cakes by shaping the mixture into small balls and gently flattening them.

Dry-fry in a non-stick frying pan until golden brown on each side.

Serve with unlimited vegetables.

Fish Curry
(Serves 4)

2 eating apples
1 large onion
15 oz (375 g) tin tomatoes
1 bay leaf
2 tablespoons oil-free sweet pickle or Branston pickle
2 tablespoons tomato purée
2 tablespoons curry powder
6 tablespoons tomato juice
2 cloves garlic, crushed
4 × 8 oz (4 × 200 g) pieces frozen haddock

Core the apples and chop them into small pieces. Finely chop the onion. Place all the ingredients except the fish in a saucepan, and bring to the boil. Cover and cook slowly for about 20 minutes, stirring occasionally.

Cut the fish into chunks and add to the mixture. Cook for a further 10 minutes.

If the mixture is too thin, remove the lid and cook on a slightly higher heat until the sauce reduces and thickens.

Serve on a bed of boiled brown rice. Allow approximately 4 oz (100 g) [cooked weight] per person.

Glazed Chicken
(Serves 4)

4 chicken breasts, part-boned, or 8 chicken thighs
1 teaspoon French mustard
3 tablespoons tomato ketchup
1 tablespoon honey
1 tablespoon soy sauce
1 tablespoon lemon juice
3/4 teaspoon ground ginger
2–3 drops Tabasco sauce
or good pinch cayenne pepper
1/2 pint (250 ml) chicken stock
1 teaspoon arrowroot
watercress
lemon wedges

Remove the skin from the chicken and make cuts in the flesh about 1/2 inch (1.25 cm) apart. Place in a shallow dish.

Mix together the mustard, tomato ketchup, honey, soy sauce, lemon juice, ground ginger and Tabasco sauce or cayenne pepper. Spoon the mixture over the chicken pieces, cover and refrigerate for 3–4 hours. Spoon the marinade over the chicken occasionally.

Remove the chicken from the dish and place in a non-stick roasting tin. Reserve the rest of the marinade. Cook the chicken in a preheated oven at 190°C, 375°F, or Gas Mark 5, for 25–30 minutes until tender. Arrange on a hot serving dish.

Stir the stock into the remainder of the marinade and mix well. Pour into a saucepan and bring to the boil. Mix the arrowroot with a little water and add to the pan. Bring to the boil again, stirring all the time.

Garnish the chicken with watercress and lemon wedges.

Serve the sauce separately.

Ham, Beef and Chicken Salad
(Serves 4)

6 oz (150 g) lean cooked ham
6 oz (150 g) lean cooked beef
2 small cooked chicken breasts
3 large oranges
2 small heads chicory
1 tablespoon white wine vinegar
or cider vinegar
3 tablespoons lemon juice
salt and black pepper
1 small lettuce
bunch watercress
1–2 tablespoons capers (optional)

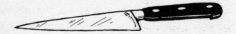

Cut the ham, beef and chicken (or turkey) into finger-length pieces.

Grate the rind and squeeze the juice from one orange. Cut the peel and pith from the other two oranges and remove the segments or cut into slices. Cut each segment into 2–3 pieces or each slice into quarters.

Wash the chicory. Reserve a few leaves and slice the rest. Mix the vinegar, orange and lemon juice together in a bowl with the grated orange rind. Season with salt and pepper.

Mix the meats, orange pieces and chicory slices together. Line a salad bowl with lettuce leaves and pour the dressing over the lettuce. Pile the meat mixture into the centre and arrange the reserved chicory spears standing up around the edge of the bowl. Garnish the top with sprigs of watercress and sprinkle a few capers over it.

Lemon Glazed Vegetables
(Serves 4)

1 lb (400 g) small new potatoes
6 oz (150 g) small new carrots
6 oz (150 g) French beans
6 oz (150 g) baby courgettes
4 oz (100 g) mange-tout
4 oz (100 g) baby sweetcorn
2^1/$_2$ oz (62.5 g) sugar
2 teaspoons French mustard
4–5 tablespoons lemon juice
grated rind of 1 lemon
1 tablespoon chopped coriander

Scrape the potatoes and carrots. Top and tail the French beans, courgettes and mange-tout. Cut each bean into 2–3 pieces. If the courgettes are very small just cut into four down the length, otherwise cut in half and then quarter them lengthways.

Cook the potatoes in a pan of boiling salted water until tender.

In another pan of boiling salted water cook the carrots for about 4 minutes, then add the French beans and cook for a further 4–5 minutes. Finally, add the courgettes, mange-tout and baby sweetcorn for a few minutes. Try to keep the vegetables slightly crisp.

Reserve about 1/4 pint (125 ml) of the mixed vegetable water and drain the rest of the vegetables. Keep hot.

Add the sugar, mustard and lemon juice to the reserved vegetable liquor and boil until syrupy.

Return the vegetables to the pan and turn carefully to coat them with the glaze. Pile into a hot serving dish and sprinkle with the grated lemon rind and the chopped coriander just before serving.

Marinated Lamb
(Serves 4–5)

4 cloves garlic
3 lbs (1.25 kg) knuckle end of leg of lamb
2 teaspoons chopped rosemary
2 teaspoons ground cumin
1 teaspoon chilli powder, or to taste
4 tablespoons red wine vinegar
1/4 pint (125 ml) red wine or cider

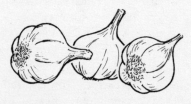

Peel the cloves of garlic. Cut 2 into slivers and crush the other two. With a small sharp knife make deep slits in the lamb and insert the slivers of garlic and some of the rosemary into each one, pressing in well with the point of the knife.

Mix together the crushed cloves of garlic, the remainder of the rosemary, the cumin and chilli powder. Stir in the vinegar, and red wine or cider.

Place the meat in a dish and pour the marinade over. Cover and keep in the refrigerator for 6–8 hours or overnight. Turn the lamb in the marinade several times so that it is well coated.

To cook, drain the meat and place in a roasting tin. Cook in a preheated oven at 180°C, 350°F, or Gas Mark 4 for about 1 1/2 hours until the meat is tender but the juices are slightly pink. If you prefer, you can remove the lamb from the oven after 1 hour, baste well with the marinade and continue cooking over a hot barbecue for a further 40–50 minutes, turning occasionally.

Mini Pizzas
(Makes 8)

This recipe will make 8 individual pizzas but if you prefer you can divide the dough and the topping into 2 and make larger pizzas for 4.

If you would rather have wholemeal bread for the base, use 10 oz (250 g) wholemeal flour and 6 oz (150 g) strong white flour.

For the base:

1 lb (400 g) packet bread flour mix
or 1 lb (400 g) strong bread flour
1 sachet easy-to-blend yeast
1 scant teaspoon salt

For the topping:

3 large onions
14 oz (350 g) tinned chopped tomatoes
1–2 cloves crushed garlic
or 1/2–1 teaspoon garlic paste
1/2 teaspoon sugar
1–2 teaspoons lemon juice
salt and black pepper
1 tablespoon chopped basil
4 oz (100 g) mushrooms
4–6 medium tomatoes
4–6 (100–150 g) ham

Prepare the bread mix for the base according to the makers' instructions. If making your own, mix the flour, yeast and salt together. Make a well in the centre and pour into it 10 fl oz (250 ml) tepid water. Blend in the flour from the sides until it is all incorporated and the dough leaves the sides of the bowl and forms a soft but not sticky ball. Knead for about 5 minutes on a lightly floured board. Return the dough to the bowl, cover with food wrap and leave in a warm place for about 1 hour until doubled in size. Meanwhile make the topping.

Peel and slice the onions and dry-fry until soft and golden brown. Remove 2–3 rounds from the pan and reserve. Add the tinned tomatoes, garlic, sugar and a little lemon juice to the pan. Season well with salt and pepper and cook over a gentle heat until the sauce mixture is quite thick. Stir in the basil.

Slice the mushrooms and tomatoes and coarsely chop the ham.

Divide the bread dough into 8 and knead each piece lightly, then roll out into a circle about the size of a saucer. Place the circles on baking sheets. Spread some of the sauce over each piece of dough. Cover with the reserved cooked onions, the ham, mushrooms and tomatoes. Leave for 15–20 minutes until the bread base has risen and bake in a preheated oven at 220°C, 425°F, or Gas Mark 7, for 12–15 minutes until the bread dough and the vegetables are cooked.

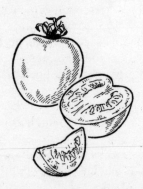

NB: If you wish, you can open freeze the pizzas at this stage. Place in a plastic bag or box. Seal the container well and store for up to 3 months. Cook from frozen, allowing an extra 5–10 minutes.

Poached Trout with Cucumber Sauce
(Serves 4)

1 carrot
1 small onion
3–4 cloves
1 bay leaf
sprig fresh thyme
a few parsley stalks
2 tablespoons white wine vinegar or cider vinegar
1/2 pint (250 ml) water
1 teaspoon salt
white pepper
4 × 8 oz (200 g) trout
1/2 cucumber, to garnish

Peel the carrot and onion. Slice the carrot thinly. Cut the onion in two and stick 2 cloves into each piece.

Place the carrot and onion in a pan with the bay leaf, fresh thyme, parsley stalks, white wine vinegar or cider vinegar and 1/2 pint (250 ml) water. Add the salt and a little white pepper and bring to the boil. Simmer gently for 20–30 minutes. This is called a *court bouillon*.

Meanwhile, scrape the scales from the trout with a small sharp knife and cut off the fins with scissors. Place in a heat-proof dish.

Pour the *court bouillon* over the fish, cover with lid and cook for 5 minutes over a gentle heat. Remove the fish carefully from the dish and take off the skins. Return the fish to the dish, replace the lid and continue cooking for another 7–8 minutes after the liquid comes to the boil. Leave in the *court bouillon* until cold.

Remove the trout from the dish and allow them to drain, then arrange on a serving dish. Finely slice the cucumber and arrange around the sides of the dish. Serve with a green salad and Cucumber Sauce (*see recipe overleaf*).

Cucumber Sauce

1/2 small cucumber
salt
1 shallot or small onion
(a pickling onion is ideal)
3–4 tablespoons lemon juice
2–3 tablespoons low-fat fromage frais
or low-fat natural yogurt
3–4 drops Tabasco sauce

Peel the cucumber and cut in half lengthways. Remove the seeds with a ball-cutter or teaspoon and cut the flesh into dice. Sprinkle with a little salt and leave for 30–40 minutes, then rinse well and spread on kitchen paper to dry.

Peel and coarsely chop the shallot or onion.

Purée the cucumber and shallot or onion in a food processor or liquidizer with lemon juice and fromage frais or yogurt.

Season to taste with Tabasco sauce and a little salt if necessary, and add more lemon juice and fromage frais or yogurt to suit your taste.

Pour into a sauceboat. Cover and chill before serving.

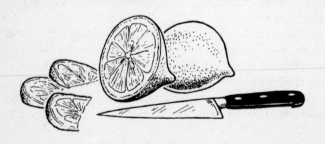

Savoury Meat Loaf
(Serves 5–6)

This dish, served cold, is ideal for a family picnic.

8 oz (200 g) lean pork
1 large onion
2 egg whites
1 lb (400 g) very lean minced beef
1 tablespoon tomato purée
1 tablespoon chopped parsley
1 tablespoon chopped chives
1 teaspoon fresh chopped thyme
or 1/4 teaspoon dried thyme
2 oz (50 g) fresh brown
or white breadcrumbs
1 1/2 teaspoons salt
black pepper

Remove any fat from the pork and peel the onion. Mince together finely.

Lightly whisk the egg whites until they are frothy.

Mix all the ingredients well together until evenly blended. Place in a 2-lb (800 g) non-stick loaf tin. Press down well and level the top with a wet tablespoon. Bake in a preheated oven at 190°C, 375°F, or Gas Mark 5, for 1–1 1/4 hours. If the juices at the side of the tin are pink, continue cooking until they are clear. Cover the top with greaseproof paper if it starts to brown too much.

Leave until cold. Turn out and slice, and serve with salad or vegetables. If you have difficulty in turning this loaf out of the tin, dip the tin in hot water for a moment or two.

You can, if you wish, serve this meat loaf hot with your favourite home-made tomato sauce or Creole Sauce (*see recipe overleaf*).

Creole Sauce

1 large onion
1–2 cloves garlic
or 1/2–1 teaspoon garlic paste
1 small green pepper
1 small red pepper
1–2 tablespoons lemon juice
1 teaspoon sugar
10 oz (250 g) tomato passata
or tinned tomatoes puréed
1 teaspoon French mustard
salt and black pepper
5 fl oz (125 ml) chicken stock, if needed
1 tablespoon chopped parsley

Peel the onion and fresh garlic. Finely chop the onion and crush the garlic. Remove the stalk, core, seeds and pith from the peppers and cut the flesh into small dice.

Place the onion, garlic, peppers, 1 tablespoon lemon juice, sugar and the tomato passata or puréed tomatoes in a pan. Stir in the French mustard and season with salt and pepper. Bring to the boil and simmer gently for 25–30 minutes until the onions and pepper are tender. If the sauce thickens too much during the cooking, add a little chicken stock whilst it is cooking, and adjust the consistency and seasoning when the sauce is cooked. Add the parsley just before serving.

This sauce is also good served with barbecued meats and fish – see **Barbecue Specials**.

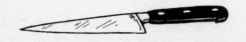

Savoury Oven-Baked Chicken Legs
(Serves 4)

8 chicken legs
2 tablespoons flour
1 teaspoon salt
1/4 teaspoon black pepper
4–6 browned breadcrumbs (*see note at end of recipe*)
1 tablespoon chopped parsley
1/2 teaspoon chopped fresh or dried rosemary
grated rind of 1 lemon
2 egg whites
2 tablespoons reduced-oil salad dressing (any brand)

Remove the skin from the chicken legs.

Combine the flour, salt and black pepper in a plastic bag.

Combine the browned breadcrumbs with the parsley, rosemary and grated lemon rind in another bag.

Whisk the egg whites until lightly frothy and mix with the reduced-oil salad dressing.

To coat the chicken legs, place one or two of them in the bag with the flour and shake until coated. Then coat them with the egg white mixture. You may find it easier to use a pastry brush to make certain they are completely coated. Shake off any surplus liquid and put them in the bag with the breadcrumbs and shake until coated. Repeat until all the chicken legs are coated.

Place in a non-stick roasting tin and bake in a pre-heated oven at 190°C, 375°F, or Gas Mark 5, for 25–30 minutes until cooked through and golden brown. Eat hot, or allow to cool and eat cold with a salad.

NB: Chicken joints and thighs can be coated in the same way, but allow an extra 5–10 minutes cooking time for chicken thighs and an extra 15 minutes for chicken pieces.

Browned breadcrumbs

Although you can use commercially made breadcrumbs, you may find that home-made ones are finer and nicer. Start by making ordinary brown or white breadcrumbs in the usual way, then place them in a thin layer in a large roasting tin. Bake them in a moderate oven until they are lightly browned, shaking the tin occasionally until they are evenly coloured. Place in a food processor or liquidizer to break down the breadcrumbs to a fine texture. If you wish, you can then sieve them to take out the coarser pieces. Return these to the food processor until they are fine. These breadcrumbs will keep for several months in an airtight container or in the freezer.

Smoked Mackerel Pâté
(Serves 3–4)

4 oz (100 g) smoked mackerel
8 oz (200 g) low-fat cottage cheese
1–2 teaspoons horseradish sauce
2 teaspoons lemon juice
salt and white pepper

Skin the mackerel and remove any bones. Break into medium-sized pieces.

Place all the ingredients in a food processor or liquidizer. If using a liquidizer, it may be advisable to purée the mixture in 2–3 batches. Purée until smooth.

Taste and add more horseradish sauce, lemon juice, salt or pepper if desired.

Turn out into a dish, cover and chill well until required.

Will serve 6 as a dinner hors d'oeuvre with 1 oz (25 g) toast per person.

Spinach and Mushroom Salad
(Serves 6–8)

4 oz (100 g) young small spinach leaves
4 oz (100 g) lamb's lettuce
1/2 bunch watercress
4 spring onions
4 oz (100 g) button mushrooms
4 tomatoes
Oil-Free Vinaigrette Dressing (*see recipe*, page 280)
nasturtium or borage flowers (optional)

Wash the spinach and lamb's lettuce well. Remove any stalks from the spinach. Wash the watercress and break into small sprigs. Trim and thinly slice the spring onions. Wipe and thinly slice the mushrooms. Peel and deseed the tomatoes and cut the flesh into strips.

Mix all the salad ingredients together in a large bowl. Pour the Oil-Free Vinaigrette Dressing over just before serving. Toss the salad and, if desired, garnish with nasturtium or borage flowers.

NB: This salad may also be used as an accompaniment to other dishes or served on its own.

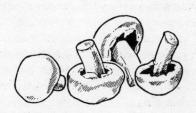

Summer Lamb Stew
(Serves 4)

3–4 small new turnips
12 small (pickling) onions
8–12 small new carrots
1 lb (400 g) small new potatoes
1¼ lbs (500 g) lean boneless lamb
½ teaspoon caster sugar
1 clove garlic or ½ teaspoon garlic paste
1½ oz (37.5 g) flour
1 pint (500 ml) lamb or chicken stock
¼ pint (125 ml) dry white wine,
cider or extra stock
1 tablespoon tomato purée
salt and black pepper
4 oz (100 g) French beans, fresh or frozen
4 oz (100 g) shelled peas, fresh or frozen
1 tablespoon mixed chopped parsley and chives

Peel the turnips and cut each into 2 or 4 pieces depending on size. Peel the onions carefully, leaving as much stem and root on as possible to prevent the centres popping out during cooking. Scrape the carrots and potatoes.

Blanch the onions in boiling salted water for 4–5 minutes and the potatoes for 7–8 minutes. Drain, then chill under cold running water. This preserves the fresh taste and the colour of the vegetables. Drain well again.

Trim any fat from the lamb. Cut the meat into 1-inch (2.5 cm) dice. Sprinkle with the sugar. Dry-fry in a frying pan or heat-proof casserole until golden brown. Remove from the pan.

Peel and crush the garlic. Mix the flour in a small bowl with a little of the stock. Whisk until smooth and add more stock. Pour into the pan with the remainder of the stock and white wine or cider, if used. Bring to the boil, stirring all the time. Add the garlic and the tomato purée. Season to taste with salt and pepper. Return the meat to a heat-proof casserole together with the turnips, onions, carrots and potatoes and bring to the boil again. Place in a preheated oven at 170°C, 325°F, or Gas Mark 3, for about 1 hour.

Top and tail fresh French beans and cut into 1-inch (2.5 cm) pieces. Blanch fresh beans and fresh peas in boiling salted water for 7–8 minutes. Drain, then chill, as before. Add to the casserole and continue cooking for about another 30 minutes until the meat and vegetables are tender. If using frozen vegetables, allow them to defrost and add to the pan 15–20 minutes before the end of cooking time.

When the meat and vegetables are tender, taste and adjust the seasoning if necessary. Pour into a hot dish or serve from the casserole. Sprinkle the parsley and chives over before serving.

Vegetable Bake
(Serves 1)

selection of vegetables e.g. carrots, parsnips,
peas, cabbage, leeks, onions
1 teaspoon mixed herbs
3 tablespoons packet stuffing mix
4 oz (100 g) mushrooms
6 oz (150 g) potato, cooked
1 cup of breadcrumbs – preferably wholemeal
1/2 pint (250 ml) vegetable stock

Wash, prepare, chop and cook the vegetables; then place them in layers in a large oven-proof dish, sprinkling the mixed herbs and stuffing mix between the layers.

Slice the mushrooms and place them over the other vegetables. Then slice the pre-cooked potato and carefully lay the slices across the top of the dish. Sprinkle the bread-crumbs on top. Carefully pour the vegetable stock over to moisten the contents of the dish.

Bake in a moderate oven (180°C, 350°F, Gas Mark 4) for 20 minutes until piping hot. Alternatively, reheat in a microwave on medium for 7 minutes and place under a hot grill for 5 minutes to crisp the top.

DESSERTS

Cheese and Apricot Pears
(Serves 4)

4 ripe pears
lemon juice
8 oz (200 g) low-fat cottage cheese
4 tablespoons apricot jam or preserve

Peel the pears, cut in half lengthways and remove the core. Brush with lemon juice to prevent discoloration.

Fill with cottage cheese mixed with apricot jam or preserve.

Serve chilled.

Gooseberry Fool
(Serves 4)

1 lb (400 g) gooseberries
2–3 oz (50–75 g) sugar
or liquid artificial sweetener to taste
green food colouring (optional)
2 meringue shells
12–16 oz (300–400 g) low-fat fromage frais
4 small sprigs mint

Top and tail the gooseberries and place in a pan with the sugar if used and 4–5 tablespoons of water. If using artificial sweetener, add after the fruit is cooked. Place over a low heat and cook gently until the fruit is barely soft. Remove and reserve a few whole gooseberries for decoration and cook the rest until they are soft.

Purée in a food processor or liquidizer. Rub through a sieve to remove the seeds and, if you wish, add a little green colouring. Cover and chill in the refrigerator.

Break the meringues into pieces and fold into the gooseberry purée. Layer the gooseberry mixture and fromage frais in tall glasses, ending with a layer of fromage frais. Decorate with the reserved gooseberries and sprigs of mint.

Refrigerate until required.

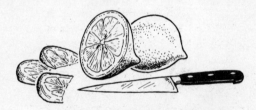

Hot Cherries and Ice Cream
(Serves 4)

15 oz (375 g) tin black cherries
3 fl oz (75 ml) cherry brandy (optional)
2 teaspoons arrowroot
4 oz (100 g) ice cream (non-Cornish variety)

Strain the cherries, reserving juice. Heat the cherry juice in a pan, add cherry brandy if desired, and thicken with enough slaked arrowroot (approximately 2 teaspoons mixed with water) to make a syrup. Stir in the cherries and pour this over 1 oz (25 g) ice cream per person.

Serve immediately.

Mango and Strawberry Bombe
(Serves 4)

2 large fresh mangoes
or 14 oz (350 g) tinned sliced mangoes
15 oz (375 g) low-fat natural yogurt
4 oz (100 g) Quark or other low-fat soft cheese
8 oz (200 g) strawberries
1–2 tablespoons lemon juice
1–2 tablespoons clear honey
2 tablespoons strawberry liqueur or Kirsch (optional)
few extra small strawberries for decoration

Set the freezer to fast freeze and chill a 2-pint (1 litre) pudding basin.

Peel the fresh mangoes and cut out the stones. If using tinned mangoes, drain well. Cut the mango flesh into large pieces.

Purée abut three-quarters of the mangoes in a food processor or liquidizer with 10 oz (250 g) of the yogurt. Place in an electric sorbet maker or in a plastic container with a lid and freeze for 2–3 hours until almost solid.

In the meantime, purée the remainder of the mangoes and yogurt with the Quark, 6 oz (150 g) of the strawberries, 1 tablespoon lemon juice, 1 tablespoon honey and the liqueur, if used, in a food processor or liquidizer until smooth. Taste and add more lemon juice and/or honey if necessary. Place in another container with a lid and freeze as before for 2–3 hours.

If the first mixture has been frozen in a plastic container, break down the ice crystals when it is almost frozen, using a food processor or an electric hand whisk. The crystals will not form if an electric sorbet-maker is used.

Place the first mixture in the chilled pudding basin and, using a large spoon, mould the ice so that it is about 1 inch (2.5 cm) thick around the sides and base of the basin. If the mixture is rather soft, fill the centre of the mould with an upright small pudding basin to keep it in place. Return it to the freezer.

Break down the crystals in the second mixture in the same way. Cut the remaining strawberries into pieces and fold into the mixture.

Remove the small basin, if used, from the ice mould. If this is firmly embedded, fill the small basin with hot water and remove immediately.

Fill the centre of the mould with the strawberry ice. Smooth over the top, cover and freeze until solid.

To serve, remove from the freezer 10–15 minutes before it is required. Dip the basin quickly into hot water and turn out on to a serving plate. Decorate with a few small strawberries.

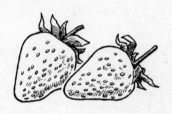

Melon with Strawberries
(Serves 4)

2 ogen or honeydew melons
8 oz (200 g) strawberries, hulled and washed

Cut the melons in half and remove all the seeds. Trim off a tiny slice of the skin at the base of each half so that they will sit securely in a dish. Fill each half with sliced strawberries.

The melons will look even better if you follow the Vandyke method when cutting them in half, by cutting jagged Vs into the side of the melon.

Melon Sundae
(Serves 4)

16 oz (400 g) melon flesh
10 oz (250 g) low-fat yogurt
(any flavour) or low-fat fromage frais
8 oz (200 g) green grapes

Finely chop the melon flesh and place in tall glasses. Spoon sufficient yogurt or fromage frais over to cover the melon. Wash, halve and seed the grapes. Divide them equally between the glasses (reserving 4 halves for decoration) and place on top of the yogurt. Add more yogurt or fromage frais on top and keep chilled until ready to serve. Decorate with 1 half-grape on top of each glass.

Minty Melon and Yogurt Salad
(Serves 4)

1 (16 oz/400 g) melon
1 stem mint
10 oz (250 g) low-fat natural yogurt
caster sugar to taste

Cut the melon in half and scoop out the seeds. Make as many melon balls as possible with a ball-cutter, or peel the melon and dice the flesh.

Wash and dry the mint. Reserve a few small sprigs for garnishing and chop the rest. Mix the yogurt and mint together and add caster sugar to taste.

Spoon the melon into the yogurt and mint mixture. Cover and refrigerate until required.

To serve, pile into individual dishes and garnish with the reserved sprigs of mint.

Pineapple, Peach and Strawberry Dessert
(Serves 4–6)

1 small pineapple or
16 oz (400 g) tinned pineapple pieces in natural juice
2 large peaches
2 tablespoons lemon juice
4 oz (100 g) white seedless grapes or 2 kiwifruit
8 oz (200 g) strawberries
6 oz (150 g) low-fat natural yogurt
2 tablespoons honey
1/4 teaspoon ground cinnamon

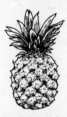

Cut the fresh pineapple in half and, using a grapefruit knife, cut out the flesh; or, if you prefer, cut the skin from the pineapple and then cut it in half. Remove the hard centre core and cut the flesh into pieces. If using tinned fruit, drain well.

Pour boiling water over the peaches and leave for 2–3 minutes. Drain and place in cold water to cool. Remove the skins and the stones and dice the flesh. Toss in the lemon juice.

Remove the stalks from the grapes or peel and slice the kiwifruit. Hull and halve the strawberries. Reserve a few grapes (or slices of kiwifruit) and a few strawberries for decoration.

Mix the yogurt, honey and cinnamon together. Add the fruit and mix well. Place in a large bowl or individual glasses. Decorate with the reserved fruit. Chill until required.

Raspberry Surprise
(Serves 6)

16 oz (400 g) frozen raspberries
4 × 5 oz (4 × 125 g) cartons
raspberry-flavoured yogurts

Thaw the raspberries slowly in the refrigerator and reserve 6 well-shaped raspberries for decoration. Place yogurt in a large bowl and gently stir in the raspberries.

Pour the mixture into stemmed wine glasses and place a raspberry on top of each. Store in the refrigerator until ready to serve.

Raspberry Yogurt Delight
(Serves 4)

2 teaspoons gelatine
1 pint (500 ml) low-fat raspberry yogurt
8 oz (200 g) raspberries
2–3 tablespoons low-fat natural
fromage frais or yogurt

Sprinkle the gelatine on to 2 tablespoons of cold water in a bowl. Leave for 4–5 minutes until soft, then stand the bowl over hot water and stir until the gelatine has dissolved. Stir the gelatine into the yogurt.

Stir 6 oz (150 g) of the raspberries into the yogurt and leave until the mixture is on the point of setting. Stir gently to ensure that the raspberries are suspended in the yogurt jelly. Pour into individual glasses and chill until set. Decorate the top of each one with a little fromage frais or yogurt and the remaining raspberries.

NB: This sweet can also be made with strawberries. In this case slice the strawberries before placing into the jelly mixture.

Red Fruit Salad
(Serves 6)

12 oz (300 g) strawberries
8 oz (200 g) raspberries
8 oz (200 g) redcurrants
4 oz (100 g) blackcurrants
4 oz (100 g) dark red cherries
4 oz (100 g) dark red plums
2–3 tablespoons sugar
or artificial sweetener to taste
2 teaspoons arrowroot
2 tablespoons Kirsch (optional)
8 oz (200 g) low-fat fromage frais
or low-fat natural yogurt
meringue fingers

Hull the strawberries and raspberries. Remove the stalks from the other fruits. Stone the cherries if desired and remove the stones from the plums. Cut the plums into ½-inch (1.25 cm) dice.

Place the redcurrants and blackcurrants in a pan with ½ pint (250 ml) water and simmer gently for 4–5 minutes until the fruit is only just tender and holds its shape. Add sugar or sweetener to taste. Mix the arrowroot with a little water and add to the pan. Bring to the boil, stirring all the time. Add the remainder of the fruit, and the Kirsh, if used, and allow to cool slightly.

Pour into a large bowl or individual bowls. Chill until required. Serve with fromage frais or yogurt, and meringue fingers.

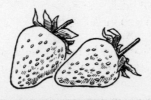

Summer Pots
(Serves 4)

1 small pineapple
or 8 oz (200 g) tinned pineapple in natural juice
8 oz (200 g) small strawberries
8 oz (200 g) blackcurrants, fresh or frozen
icing sugar or artificial sweetener to taste
low-fat natural fromage frais or yogurt, to serve

Cut the skin from the pineapple, then cut in half and remove the hard centre core. Dice the rest of the pineapple, or drain the tinned pineapple. Wash and hull the strawberries and mix with the pineapple. Place the fruit in 4 dishes.

Remove the stalks from fresh blackcurrants. Cook in a scant 5 fl oz (125 ml) water until tender. Purée very lightly in a food processor or liquidizer (only enough to break down the fruit – take care not to purée the seeds). Rub the blackcurrant mixture through a sieve to remove the seeds. Add icing sugar or sweetener to taste.

Pour the blackcurrant purée over the pineapple and strawberries just before serving.

Serve topped with fromage frais or yogurt.

BARBECUE SPECIALS

Assorted kebabs: The cooking times given are appropriate for a preheated barbecue.

Small onions are very tasty with kebabs, but as onions need longer cooking prepare them first. Pickling onions are also ideal.

Peel the onions carefully, leaving as much of the stem and stalk on as possible to prevent the insides popping out while they are cooking. Blanch in boiling salted water for 5–7 minutes. Drain, chill under cold running water, drain well again and use as required.

Barbecue Sauce
(Serves 2)

3 tablespoons tomato ketchup
3 tablespoons brown sauce
1 teaspoon mustard (English or French)
2 tablespoons garlic and chilli sauce
6 tablespoons tomato juice
1 clove garlic, crushed (optional)
freshly ground black pepper

Mix all the ingredients together and brush on to the
kebabs, meat or poultry, preferably an hour or two before
cooking. Heat any remaining sauce and serve separately.

Beef and Mushroom Kebabs
(Serves 4)

1 lb (400 g) very thin slices topside beef
or rump steak
8 small onions
8 small mushrooms

Cut the beef into 16 pieces. Prepare the onions as described
above and wrap each onion and mushroom in a piece of
beef.

Thread four beef rolls on to each skewer. Cooking time
approximately 7–10 minutes.

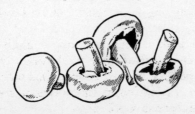

Kidney and Tomato Kebabs
(Serves 4)

4 lamb's kidneys
4 rashers lean bacon
1–2 green peppers
8 small tomatoes

Cut the kidneys in half, remove any membrane and the cores and soak in cold, lightly salted water for 30 minutes.

Stretch the bacon with a knife and cut each rasher in two. Roll up.

Remove the core, seeds and pith from the peppers and cut into 8 pieces.

Drain the kidneys well and thread all the ingredients alternately on to the skewers. Cooking time approximately 5–7 minutes.

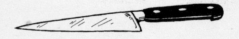

Lamb and Mushroom Kebabs
(Serves 4)

1 lb (400 g) lean boneless lamb
1–2 red peppers
4 small tomatoes
8 small mushrooms
4 bay leaves

Cut the lamb into 1-inch (2.5 cm) pieces.

Remove the core, seeds and pith from the peppers and cut into 8 pieces.

Thread the lamb, peppers, tomatoes, mushrooms and bay leaves alternately on to the skewers. Cooking time approximately 10 minutes.

Liver and Bacon Kebabs
(Serves 4)

12 oz (300 g) lamb's liver in one piece
a little milk
8 small onions
4–6 oz (100–150 g) bacon steak
2–3 tablespoons lemon juice
8 small mushrooms
3–4 tablespoons fresh breadcrumbs

Cut the liver into 1-inch (2.5 cm) pieces and soak in the milk for 20–30 minutes. Drain well. Prepare the onions as described previously.

Cut the bacon into 1-inch (2.5 cm) squares. Sprinkle the lemon juice over the mushrooms and toss the liver, bacon and mushrooms in the breadcrumbs.

Thread all the ingredients on to the skewers. Cooking time approximately 5–7 minutes.

Pork and Apricot Kebabs
(Serves 4)

1 lb (400 g) lean boneless pork
8 oz (200 g) tin apricot halves in natural juice
8 small onions
8 bay leaves

Cut the pork into 1-inch (2.5 cm) pieces. Drain the apricots and prepare the onions as described previously.

Thread the meat, apricots, onions and bay leaves alternately on to the skewers. Cooking time approximately 12–15 minutes.

Surf 'n' Turf
(Serves 4)

16 large prawns without heads, peeled
12 oz (300 g) fillet or rump steak
4 limes or 2 lemons
1 onion or a few spring onions
1 clove garlic or ½ teaspoon garlic paste
salt
freshly ground black pepper

Wash and thoroughly drain the peeled prawns. Cut the steak into 1–inch (2.5 cm) cubes and place in a shallow dish with the prawns.

Grate the rind and squeeze the juice from 3 of the limes or 1 of the lemons. Cut the remaining lime or lemon into four and reserve.

Peel the onion or trim the spring onions. Peel and crush the garlic, finely chop the onion or shred the spring onions. Mix together with the lime or lemon juice and rind and season with salt and black pepper. Pour over the meat and prawns. Cover and leave in the refrigerator for about 2 hours, turning the meat and prawns occasionally in the marinade.

Thread the meat and prawns alternately on to the skewers and cook over a preheated barbecue or under a preheated grill for 8–10 minutes. Serve with the remaining lime or lemon quarters.

Tomato and Courgette Kebabs
(Serves 4)

1 lb (400 g) courgettes
1–2 tablespoons lemon juice
8 small onions
8 small tomatoes

Trim the courgettes and cut into 1-inch (2.5 cm) pieces. Blanch in boiling salted water for about 2 minutes. Drain and chill under cold running water. Drain again and sprinkle the lemon juice over. Prepare the onions as described previously.

Thread the courgettes, onions and tomatoes alternately on to the skewers. Cooking time approximately 10 minutes.

Assorted meat and poultry dishes

The following recipes can be easily adapted for an outdoor barbecue. Always ensure that the meat or poultry is thoroughly cooked on all sides and allow sufficient time for the sauces and marinades to be prepared in advance.

Barbecued Chicken/Drumsticks
(Serves 4)

2 medium-sized onions
1 clove fresh garlic or 1/2 teaspoon garlic paste
14 oz (350 g) tin tomatoes
2 tablespoons Worcestershire sauce
1 tablespoon honey
1 teaspoon paprika
salt and freshly ground black pepper
4 chicken quarters or 8 drumsticks
1/2 bunch watercress or parsley, to garnish

Any cut of chicken can be barbecued in this way. Drumsticks are ideal, or you could use this recipe as an alternative way of preparing poussins. If you prefer, you can cook the chicken in a preheated oven (200°C, 400°F, Gas Mark 6) for 35–40 minutes.

To make the sauce, peel the onions and fresh garlic. Finely chop the onions and crush the garlic. Place in a pan with the tomatoes (including their juice), Worcestershire sauce, honey and paprika. Season to taste with salt and freshly ground black pepper. Bring to the boil and simmer, uncovered, for 30 minutes until the onions are tender and the sauce has thickened slightly.

Remove all skin and fat from the chicken. Brush well with the sauce and cook over a preheated barbecue or under a preheated hot grill for 25–30 minutes. The cooking time will depend on the thickness of the flesh – chicken quarters will take longer than drumsticks. Turn them once or twice during cooking, and brush with more sauce. To make certain the chicken is cooked, prick the flesh with a fork. When the juices run clear, it is cooked.

Garnish with watercress or parsley just before serving the dish hot, with the remaining sauce served separately.

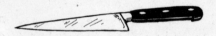

Barbecued Pork Pouches
(Serves 4)

1 small onion
1 clove fresh garlic or 1/2 teaspoon garlic paste
2–3 oz (50–75 g) mushrooms
1–2 teaspoons curry powder
3 tablespoons tomato purée
salt
freshly ground black pepper
2 tablespoons fresh breadcrumbs
4 × 5–6 oz (4 × 125–150 g) lean loin pork chops
1/2 teaspoon cinnamon
1/4 teaspoon ground cloves
good pinch nutmeg
1 teaspoon brown sugar
10 fl oz (250 ml) cider
1 teaspoon arrowroot

Peel the onion and garlic. Finely chop the onion and crush the garlic. Dry-fry the onion and half the garlic in a pre-heated frying pan until they are almost soft.

Trim and finely chop the mushrooms. Add to the pan and continue cooking until the mushrooms are soft and the mixture is dry. Remove from the heat, then stir in the curry powder and 1 tablespoon of the tomato purée. Season well with salt and pepper, then stir in the breadcrumbs.

Trim all the fat from the chops and make a deep slit in the side of each right up to the bone to form a large pocket. Divide the mushroom and onion mixture into 4 and place a portion in each pocket. Press well in and press the edges together to seal in the mixture.

Mix the remainder of the garlic and tomato purée in a flat dish and stir in the cinnamon, ground cloves, nutmeg and brown sugar. Season lightly with salt and pepper and moisten with half the cider. Place the chops in the marinade and coat them well. Leave for 1–2 hours, turning occasionally.

Drain the marinade from each chop and reserve. Cook the chops over a preheated barbecue or under a preheated grill for 8–10 minutes on each side or until the meat looks cooked down the centre of the bone.

Meanwhile mix the remainder of the marinade and cider together. Make this up to 10 fl oz (250 ml) with water and place in a small pan and bring to the boil. Mix the arrowroot with a little cold water and add to the pan. Bring to the boil again, stirring all the time and then check the seasoning. Serve with the cooked chops.

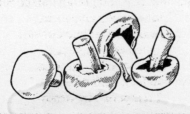

Beefburgers
(Makes approximately 16)

2 lbs (800 g) lean beef
or finely minced lean beef
2 large onions
1–2 cloves garlic
4 oz (100 g) stale bread
2 egg whites
1 teaspoon French mustard
1/4 teaspoon allspice
1/2 teaspoon mixed dried herbs
2 teaspoons salt
black pepper

Mince the beef very finely by passing it through a mincer 2–3 times. If using bought mince, make certain it is very fresh.

Peel the onions and garlic. Chop the onion very finely and crush the garlic, or put them both into a food processor until they are almost puréed.

Soak the bread in a little water for about 5 minutes, then squeeze out the liquid.

Whisk the egg whites until frothy.

In a large bowl mix all the ingredients together. It is easier to use your hands for this. If you wish to check the seasoning, dry-fry a small portion of the mixture in a pre-heated non-stick frying-pan, and taste.

Form the beefburgers either in a mould or by shaping them with wet hands. Layer them with a piece of freezer tissue between each, and store in a plastic box in the freezer. They can then be removed separately.

Dry-fry, grill or cook over a preheated barbecue as required. They will take about 4–5 minutes to cook on each side. Frozen beefburgers need a minute or two longer than fresh ones.

Spicy Pork Steaks
(Serves 4)

1½ teaspoons cayenne pepper
1 teaspoon ground ginger
4 teaspoons cornflour
1 tablespoon Canderel
4 teaspoons tomato purée
2 cloves fresh garlic, crushed
1 pint (500 ml) cold water
1 beef stock cube, crumbled
4 pork steaks, fat removed
(approximately 4 oz [100 g] each without bone)

Place all the dry ingredients in a non-stick pan with the tomato purée and crushed garlic. Add a little of the water to make a thin paste. Slowly add the remaining water and the stock cube. Bring to the boil, stirring continuously. Remove from the heat and allow to cool.

Score the surface of the pork steaks and place them in a shallow dish. With a pastry brush, paint some of the cold sauce on both sides of the pork steaks and leave to marinate for an hour or so.

When ready to cook the steaks, place them on a rack and paint again with more sauce. Cook over a preheated barbecue or under a grill at medium heat. After 5 minutes, turn the steaks over and paint with more sauce. Keep turning them until they are crisp and brown on both sides (approximately 30 minutes). Heat any remaining sauce for serving with the steaks.

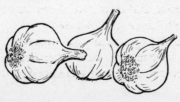

Assorted salads: The following salads are ideal for a barbecue party and can be served either as side dishes or as main course alternatives.

Courgette and Tomato Salad
(Serves 4)

2 small heads chicory
4 tomatoes
2 courgettes
1 bunch radishes
5 oz (125 g) low-fat fromage frais or yogurt
1/2 teaspoon French mustard
1 tablespoon chopped gherkins
or 1 tablespoon chopped spring onions
1 tablespoon chopped parsley
salt and pepper

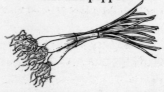

Wash the chicory. Reserve a few leaves for garnishing and slice the rest. Skin and seed the tomatoes and chop the flesh coarsely. Trim the courgettes, cut into 2–3 pieces and slice lengthways, then cut into matchstick-sized pieces. Coarsely grate half the radishes and slice the rest.

Mix together the fromage frais or yogurt, French mustard, the gherkins or spring onions, and chopped parsley. Season to taste.

Mix the sliced chicory, tomatoes, courgettes and grated radishes together. Fold in the sauce and pile the salad on to a dish. Garnish each end of the dish with the reserved leaves of chicory. Arrange the sliced radishes down the side of the dish. Chill until required.

Cucumber and Strawberry Salad
(Serves 4–6)

1 small cucumber
6–8 oz (150–200 g) strawberries
1 tablespoon white wine vinegar
salt and black pepper

Peel the cucumber and slice thinly. Slice the strawberries
from top to bottom. Arrange the cucumber and strawberry
slices in alternate rings on a plate. Sprinkle the vinegar over
and season.

Cucumber Boats with Tuna
(Serves 4)

This dish is suitable as an hors d'oeuvre for a dinner party
or as a barbecue side dish. It can also be made with tinned
salmon.

1 cucumber
2 whites of hard-boiled eggs
8 oz (200 g) tinned tuna in brine
4 oz (100 g) Quark or other low-fat soft cheese
or cottage cheese
1 teaspoon made-up mustard
1 tablespoon lemon juice
1 tablespoon chopped parsley
1 tablespoon chopped chives or spring onions
salt and pepper
a few lettuce leaves

Peel the cucumber, cut off the ends and cut in half. Then
slice each half in two lengthways. Remove the seeds with a
ball-cutter or teaspoon and discard. Blanch the cucumber
shells in boiling salted water for 3–5 minutes. Drain and

chill under cold running water. Drain well again, then dry on kitchen paper.

Chop the egg whites and keep to one side.

Drain the tuna fish and, using a fork, mash together with the Quark, low-fat cheese or cottage cheese and the mustard and lemon juice. If you prefer a smoother mixture, purée the fish and other ingredients in a food processor or liquidizer. Stir in most of the parsley, and chives or spring onions, and season to taste.

Fill the cucumber shells with the mixture and arrange on a lettuce-covered dish or individual plates. Sprinkle the chopped egg whites and remaining herbs over the top. Chill in the refrigerator until required.

Niçoise Salad
(Serves 4)

12 oz (300 g) new potatoes
8 oz (200 g) French beans
4 medium-sized tomatoes
8 oz (200 g) tinned tuna fish in brine
4 anchovy fillets (optional)
2–3 tablespoons Oil-Free Vinaigrette Dressing
(*see recipe*, page 280)
1 small lettuce
a few capers (optional
1–2 hard-boiled eggs

Scrape the new potatoes and cook in boiling salted water until tender. Drain and chill under cold running water. Drain well again and slice or dice the potatoes.

Top and tail the French beans and cut each one into 2–3 pieces. Cook in boiling salted water for 8–10 minutes until only just tender. Chill and drain as above.

Peel the tomatoes and cut into quarters. Drain the tuna fish and break into chunks. Wash the anchovy fillets in cold water and cut in half lengthways.

Mix together the potatoes, French beans, tomatoes, tuna fish and the Oil-Free Vinaigrette.

Line a dish or bowl with lettuce leaves. Pile the mixture in the centre. Garnish the top with the strips of anchovy, if used. Sprinkle the capers over the top and arrange thin wedges of egg around the outside of the fish mixture. Cover and refrigerate until required.

Oriental Prawn Salad
(Serves 6)

6 oz (150 g) easy-to-cook rice
1 fish stock cube (optional)
2 oz (50 g) mixed red and green peppers, chopped
2 oz (50 g) cooked peas
2 oz (50 g) cooked sweetcorn
4 tablespoons Oil-Free Vinaigrette Dressing
(*see recipe*, page 280)
salt and pepper
1 small cucumber
4 tomatoes
1/2 bunch spring onions
5oz (125g) low-fat natural yogurt
2 tablespoons tomato ketchup
1–2 teaspoons curry powder
1 small lettuce
1–11/2 lbs (400–600 g) prawns
4–6 whole prawns

Rinse the rice and cook with the stock cube according to the instructions on the packet. Leave until cold then mix with the peppers, peas, sweetcorn and the Oil-Free Vinaigrette. Season to taste if necessary and arrange in a ring around the sides of a flat dish.

Meanwhile, cut off one-quarter of the cucumber and reserve. Peel the remaining three-quarters and slice in half lengthways. Remove the seeds with a ball-cutter or teaspoon and cut the flesh into small dice. Sprinkle a little salt over and leave for about 30 minutes, then rinse and drain well.

Peel and deseed one tomato. Cut into dice. Thinly slice the remainder of the cucumber and tomatoes. Cut each slice in half. Trim and thinly slice the spring onions.

Mix together the yogurt and tomato ketchup and curry powder to taste. Season well.

Wash the lettuce and drain well. Garnish each end of the dish with lettuce and finely shred the rest.

Make certain the prawns are completely defrosted. Rinse and drain them well. Mix together with the shredded lettuce, diced cucumber, diced tomato and spring onions. Stir in the yogurt mixture and check the seasoning. Remove the shells from the tails of the whole prawns, leaving the heads intact.

Pile the prawn mixture into the centre of the rice. Arrange half slices of tomato and cucumber alternately around the dish, and place the whole prawns in the centre. Cover and refrigerate until required.

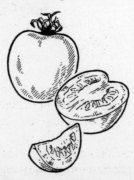

Potato Salad
(Serves 4)

1 lb (400 g) new potatoes
5 oz (125 g) natural yogurt
4 fl oz (100 ml) reduced-oil salad dressing,
e.g. Waistline
salt and pepper to taste

Scrape the new potatoes and cook in boiling salted water until tender. Drain and chill under cold running water. Drain again and dice the potatoes, then mix with all the other ingredients.

Prawn and Pasta Salad
(Serves 4)

1 lb (400 g) cooked medium-sized pasta shells
1 lb (400 g) prawns, peeled, de-veined, and cooked
5 oz (125 g) natural yogurt
1 tablespoon tomato purée
few drops Tabasco sauce to taste
3 spring onions

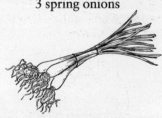

Combine the pasta shells and prawns in a serving bowl.

In a small bowl, stir together the yogurt, tomato purée and Tabasco sauce. Pour on to the pasta mixture and toss well.

Sprinkle with finely chopped spring onions just before serving at room temperature or very slightly chilled.

Rosy Duck Salad
(Serves 4–6)

4$\frac{1}{2}$ lbs (1.8 kg) cold roasted duck
2 oranges
5 tablespoons low-fat fromage frais
2 tablespoons tomato ketchup
1–2 teaspoons curry powder
1 teaspoon French mustard
salt and white pepper
6–8 very small tomatoes
1 pink grapefruit
$\frac{1}{2}$ small red pepper
$\frac{1}{2}$ small yellow pepper
a small selection of red salads,
e.g. $\frac{1}{2}$ lollo rosso, $\frac{1}{2}$ oak-leaved lettuce,
plus a little raddichio
a few nasturtium flowers (optional)

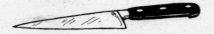

Remove the skin from the duck and cut the meat into small strips.

Grate the rind from one orange. Remove the rind from the other, the pith from both oranges and cut out the segments. Mix the duck with the orange segments and grated rind.

Mix the fromage frais with the tomato ketchup, curry powder and mustard. Season and carefully fold about half into the duck and the orange segments.

Wash the tomatoes. Cut the peel and pith from the grapefruit and cut out the segments. Remove the core, pith and seeds from the peppers and cut into thin strips.

Arrange some of the red-leaved salad on a serving dish. Pile the duck and orange mixture in the centre and garnish with the grapefruit segments, 3–4 tomatoes, a few strips of pepper and the nasturtium flowers, if used. Serve the rest of the salad in a separate bowl. Also serve the rest of the sauce separately. Refrigerate until required.

Sweetcorn and Red Bean Salad
(Serves 2)

16 oz (400 g) tin red kidney beans
2 × 12 oz (2 × 300 g) tins sweetcorn niblets

Drain and wash the kidney beans, then mix together with the sweetcorn niblets.

Serve on a dish.

Three Bean Salad
(Serves 4)

15 oz (375 g) tin red kidney beans,
15 oz (375 g) tin haricot beans,
8 oz (200 g) tin butter beans,
1 cucumber
3 tomatoes
4 sticks celery
8 spring onions
1 red or green pepper
1 Spanish onion
sprinkling of oregano and sage
salt and freshly ground black pepper

Drain and wash the kidney, haricot and butter beans. Finely chop the cucumber, tomatoes, celery, spring onions, red or green pepper and Spanish onion.

Mix all the ingredients together in a large bowl. Season to taste.

Serve chilled.

Tomato and Cucumber Salad
(Serves 4)

6 firm tomatoes
$1/2$ cucumber
6 spring onions
freshly ground black pepper
pinch of salt

Cut tomatoes into wedge-shaped pieces. Peel the cucumber, then slice in half lengthways and deseed with a ball-cutter or teaspoon. Chop the cucumber flesh into cubes. Finely chop the spring onions.

Mix all the ingredients together in a bowl and season to taste.

Serve chilled.

CAKES

Banana and Sultana Cake
(1 serving = $1/2$–inch/1.25 cm slice)

1 lb 3 oz (475 g) ripe bananas (5 large peeled)
2 eggs
6 oz (150 g) brown sugar
4 oz (100 g) sultanas
8 oz (200 g) self-raising flour

Mash bananas and add eggs, sugar and sultanas. Mix well, then stir in the flour. Place in a lined 2-lb (800 g) loaf tin or cake tin.

Bake for $1 1/4$ hours in a preheated oven at 180°C, 350°F, Gas Mark 4. Store in an airtight tin for 24 hours before serving.

This can be an economical recipe as very ripe bananas can often be purchased cheaply.

Kim's Cake
(1 serving = 1/2-inch/1.25 cm slice)

1 lb (400 g) dried mixed fruit
1 mug hot black tea
1 mug soft brown sugar
2 mugs self-raising flour
1 beaten egg

Soak the dried fruit overnight in the black tea. The next day, mix all the ingredients (including the tea) together, then place into a 2-lb (800 g) loaf tin or round cake tin. Bake for 2 hours at 160°C, 325°F, or Gas Mark 3.

To make into a birthday-type fruit cake, add some cherries to the dried fruit.

This cake can be frozen.

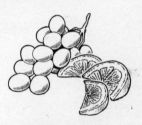

DRESSINGS

Garlic Dressing

1 clove garlic
5 oz (125 g) low-fat natural yogurt
1 tablespoon wine vinegar
1 tablespoon reduced-oil salad dressing (any brand)
salt and freshly ground black pepper

Crush the garlic and then mix all the ingredients together. Store in a screw-top jar in the refrigerator and use within 2 days.

Oil-Free Vinaigrette Dressing

3 tablespoons white wine vinegar or cider vinegar
1 tablespoon lemon juice
1/2 teaspoon black pepper
1/2 teaspoon salt
1 teaspoon sugar
1/2 teaspoon French mustard
chopped herbs (thyme, marjoram, basil or parsley)

Mix all the ingredients together. Place in a container, seal and shake well. Taste, and add more salt or sugar as desired.

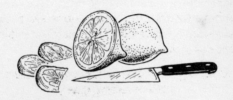

Marie Rose Dressing

2 tablespoons tomato ketchup
1 tablespoon reduced-oil salad dressing (any brand)
dash Tabasco sauce
squeeze lemon juice

Mix all ingredients together well and store in a screw-top jar in the refrigerator until needed.

Reduced-Oil Salad Dressing

Mix 3 tablespoons reduced-oil low-calorie salad dressing (any brand) with 5 oz (125 g) plain low-fat yogurt. Add salt and pepper to taste.
Keep in a refrigerator for up to 2 days.

DRINKS

Summer sunshine calls for delicious thirst-quenchers that don't contain too many calories. Here are some of my favourites.

Apple Cola

Mix a can of diet cola with one can of Appletize.
Serve in a tall glass with ice.

Buck's Fizz

This drink is for special summer occasions and to celebrate the new slimline you after following the 14–day Shape-Up for Summer diet and exercise programme.

freshly squeezed orange juice, well chilled
1 bottle champagne
or 1 bottle dry, white, sparkling wine, well chilled

Fill champagne flutes or wineglasses one-third full with orange juice. Top up with champagne or sparkling white wine. Cheers!

Caribbean Surprise

5 fl oz (125 ml) unsweetened pineapple juice
slimline ginger ale

Mix in a tall glass with plenty of ice. Top up with ginger ale as desired.
Garnish with a cherry, pineapple and orange slices and pineapple or mint leaves on a cocktail stick.

Grapefruit Fizz

4 oz (100 ml) unsweetened grapefruit juice
slimline tonic water

Pour the unsweetened grapefruit juice into a tall glass and add plenty of ice. Add the slimline tonic to taste, and top up with the remainder of the tonic when required.

This drink is an excellent 'filler' before a meal.

Pineapple Sludge

5 fl oz (125 ml) unsweetened pineapple juice
1 can diet cola

Half fill a glass with ice, pour the pineapple juice over and top up with the diet cola. Although the appearance of the drink may be off-putting, the taste is delicious.

St Clements

slimline orange
slimline bitter lemon

Pour half a bottle of each into a tall glass with plenty of ice. Top up as required.

For an extra special drink, use freshly squeezed orange juice with the bitter lemon.

Pacific Delight

3 fl oz (75 ml) low-calorie lime cordial
low-calorie ginger ale

Pour the lime cordial into a tall glass with plenty of ice and top it with the ginger ale to taste.

Sangria
(Serves 4–8)

Any selection of fruit can be used in addition to the orange and lemons. Try a few pieces of melon or a kiwifruit instead of the peach or, when fruit is expensive, just use the basic lemon and orange ingredients.

2 lemons
1 orange
1 peach
2–3 oz (50–75 g) strawberries
1 bottle red wine
1–2 tablespoons sugar (optional)
1 pint (500 ml) slimline lemonade

Squeeze the juice from one lemon and thinly slice the other lemon and the orange. Cut the slices in half.

Pour boiling water over the peach. Leave for a minute or two, then place in cold water to chill. Remove the skin and the stone and thinly slice the flesh. Toss the peach slices in the lemon juice. Hull and slice the strawberries.

Place the fruit and lemon juice in a large jug and add the red wine. Sweeten to taste if desired. Chill until required.

Just before serving add the lemonade and a few ice cubes.

Sludge Gulper

4 fl oz (100 ml) unsweetened orange juice
1 can diet cola

Pour the orange juice into a tall glass with plenty of ice. Add the diet cola to taste.

Serve with a straw.

Spritzer

5 fl oz (125 ml) white wine
sparkling mineral water or soda water

Pour the wine into a large-sized wineglass and add the mineral water or soda water. This makes a long and very enjoyable drink that can accompany a meal or be drunk pleasurably on its own.

Summer Punch
(Serves 4–8)

1 lb (400 g) strawberries
icing sugar, to taste
1 bottle white wine, chilled
soda water or slimline lemonade
a few sprigs mint

Wash and hull the strawberries. Slice 6 to 8 of the strawberries and purée the rest in a food processor or liquidizer; then sieve to remove the seeds. Sweeten to taste with icing sugar. Chill the purée.

Mix the white wine with the strawberry purée. Half fill glasses with the mixture. Add a few sliced strawberries and a couple of ice cubes and top up with soda water or slimline lemonade. Garnish each glass with a sprig of mint.

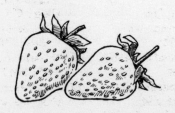

INDEX OF RECIPES